MW01489623

The Ultimate Guide to Autistic Burnout

Evidence-based information empowering autistics & clinicians to better understand and assist those with autistic burnout

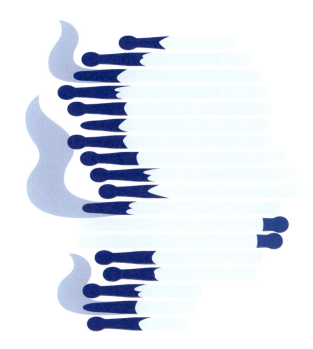

Dr. Natalie Engelbrecht ND RP
Dr. Debra Bercovici PhD
Eva Silvertant BDes & Kendall Jones

Illustrations by Eva Silvertant

Researched, written, and edited by autistics.

Dr. Natalie Engelbrecht, ND, MSc, RP, a late-diagnosed autistic health care professional for autistic adults and teens.

Dr. Debra Bercovici, PhD, a late-diagnosed AuDHDer and Assistant Professor, Teaching Stream at the University of Toronto Scarborough.

Eva Silvertant, BDes, a late-diagnosed AuDHDer and a writer, researcher, and art director for Embrace Autism.

Kendall Jones, a late-diagnosed AuDHDer and a writer/editor for Embrace Autism.

Design & illustrations by **Eva Silvertant**.
Additional edits by **Hailey Revolone**.

→ Last revised: November 14, 2024

Embrace Autism's 'The Ultimate Guide to' series
The constructs in this book series are often not included in health-care providers' curricula. This series aims to offer evidence-based and current information to guide autistic individuals, their caregivers, and healthcare providers toward autism-affirming approaches.

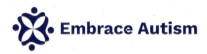

Introduction

As a clinician and someone diagnosed with autism later in life, searching for self-understanding, I felt frustrated by the scarcity of reliable information.

I discovered that many clinicians have little if any training on autism in people without intellectual or language disabilities, even though this group represents the majority of autistic individuals, accounting for **66%** (Shenouda et al, 2023).

This book endeavours to address some of those clinical blind spots, and provides accessible information for busy practitioners and non-professionals alike.

Aim of the Book

Here, we construct a comprehensive and evidence-based account of autistic burnout by combining current lines of research with clinical experience, the lived experience of autistic people with autistic burnout, and theoretical approaches; and the invaluable insights shared by autistic individuals.

In our guidebooks, the expertise of autistic individuals is valued equally to evidence-based approaches. This serves to fill an existing gap in clinician knowledge about autism (McCormack et al., 2020).

With that, the aim of this book has been to provide a resource that allows for more patient autonomy and better clinical understanding—as well as to facilitate a beneficial patient–doctor relationship.

With this book we endeavour to foster informed discussions and educate healthcare professionals and non-professionals with evidence-based information, so that autistic people can be better understood and treated.

Language Used

In this book, we choose autism-affirming language for clinicians and laypersons. The way we talk about autism continues to evolve. The majority of autistics prefer identity-first language; we refer to people as 'autistic' rather than 'people with autism.'

When we speak of autism, we also refer to autistics with co-occurring Attention Deficit Hyperactivity Disorder (ADHD)—colloquially known as 'AuDHD'.

Autism Research

Adult autism research is still disproportionately lacking. For instance, a 2017 review of the literature estimated that only **3.5%** of published research on autism focused on adults of any age (Howlin & Magiati, 2017); and only **3%** of U.S. autism research funds in 2018 went to study people "as they progress into and through adulthood" (Autism Research Database, 2018). It is also important to note that studies on autistic people of colour are severely lacking; and there is a similar gap in autistic gender-based research.

Much of the autism research is likely blended with AuDHD because, before 2013, the belief was that autism and ADHD could not co-occur; it wasn't until 2013 that the DSM acknowledged that autism and ADHD could co-occur, and clinicians took even longer to adapt due to what they had previously learned. Yet according to the scientific literature, an estimated **60–70%** percent of autistic also meet the criteria for ADHD (Eaton et al., 2023); and conversely, **20–50%** of people with ADHD meet the criteria for autism (Rommelse et al., 2010).

The Subjects of This Book

Not all autistic individuals or groups represent the entire autistic community. This book does not center on the **33%** of autistic individuals who are nonverbal or have intellectual disabilities. Additionally, it does not focus on children.

We recognize that there is a segment of the autistic population that needs ongoing care and support and is more likely to receive an autism diagnosis. We want to acknowledge and respect the experiences of these individuals and their loved ones. Please keep in mind that they are not the focus of this book.

About Embrace Autism

In 2018, Eva Silvertant and I, Dr. Natalie Engelbrecht, ND, RP—both late-diagnosed autistics—co-founded Embrace Autism. Our mission has been to provide research and experience-based information on autism for adults.

We believe that quality information can empower us and our fellow autistics by helping us understand and appreciate ourselves, discover our incredible potential, and acknowledge the beauty and splendour in ourselves and each other.

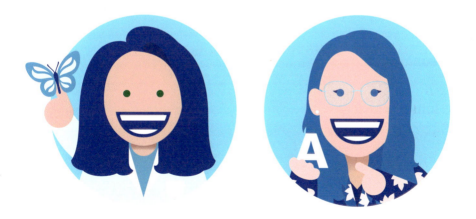

Visit our website at Embrace-Autism.com

Overview

About This Book

This book has two sections: one for healthcare providers—written using clinical terminology—and another for those unfamiliar with medical jargon. It emphasizes the importance of involving patients in their healthcare and acknowledges their expertise—because who knows you better than yourself?

The clinical and non-clinical sections contain unique information targeted toward the intended reader.

	Clinical	Non-clinical
Language:	Clinical	Accessible
Content:	For clinical use	For personal use
Descriptions:	Brevity	Comprehensive explanations
Papers referenced:	APA-style citations	Footnotes
Personal examples:	—	√
Links to articles:	—	√

Clinical Version

The clinical version is placed first to provide easy access to busy healthcare providers. It provides a reference for healthcare providers to guide clinical decision-making by providing unbiased, evidence-based, practical information on autistic burnout. It aims to provide concise information so that practitioners can competently assess, diagnose, and treat autistic burnout—as well as better understand and communicate with their autistic patients as a whole.

There will always be a complex inter-communication problem between autistics and their healthcare providers (the double or triple empathy problem), which works both ways; autistics have difficulty understanding how to explain their symptoms, and healthcare providers have difficulty understanding what autistic people intend to communicate. This is a barrier for autistic patients to receive optimum care. The clinical section includes information on how to overcome this barrier.

Non-Clinical Version

The non-clinical section translates medical to non-medical language to allow autistics and their loved ones to be part of their healthcare team. Patients have the right to autonomy, which can only be achieved by fully understanding themselves and the options available. To this end, the non-clinical section includes a step-by-step approach to navigating a healthcare visit, aiming to clarify an often intimidating situation.

The non-clinical version includes examples, personal anecdotes from autistic people with autistic burnout, and additional information and links to external sources—including articles from our website (each containing references to more research papers)—that may be useful both to autistic people and for medical practitioners should they desire a deeper understanding.

About the Authors

Dr. Natalie Engelbrecht, ND, RP

A late-diagnosed (46) autistic cis-female

Dr. Natalie Engelbrecht is a naturopathic doctor and registered psychotherapist with a focus on adult autism without intellectual disability. She is a highly accomplished and widely respected clinician with a special interest in Autism Spectrum Disorder (ASD).

She has nearly 30 years of experience in private practice and is the co-founder of Embrace Autism—an internationally renowned website that provides research and experience-based information on autism.

Natalie holds a degree in Psychology from McMaster University, a Master's with distinction in Applied Clinical Psychology from the University of Liverpool, and a Doctor of Naturopathy degree.

Her work has significantly contributed to the global understanding of autism.

Dr. Debra Bercovici, PhD

A late-diagnosed (28) BIPOC cis-female with ADHD

Dr. Debra Bercovici is an Assistant Professor Teaching Stream at the University of Toronto Scarborough, where she teaches Neuroscience and Psychology.

She completed her doctorate at the University of British Columbia in Behavioural Neuroscience, investigating the neurocircuitry underlying executive functioning. Currently, her research has shifted to understanding the experiences of marginalized students in university, including autistic students.

Debra is also in the process of completing a Master of Arts in Counselling Psychology degree.

Starting in September 2024, she will be offering individual therapy for fellow neurodivergent, disabled, racialized, and LGBTQIA+ adults looking to process trauma and explore their identity through a justice-oriented lens.

Eva Silvertant, BDes
A late-diagnosed (25) trans-female with ADHD

Eva Silvertant is a co-founder of Embrace Autism, and is living up to her name as a silver award-winning graphic designer.

She has a degree in multi-media design and a BA in graphic design, with 22 years of experience as a graphic designer and illustrator—having launched her freelance design/art career at the age of 13. She has worked for a myriad of brands and clients from various industries and disciplines, and had her work published in books and magazines, and won several awards for graphic and type design.

She specializes in communication at various levels, from writing and sharing knowledge to communication through design, typography, and type design. A lifelong learner with an insatiable thirst for knowledge and an affinity for synthesizing research, she is particularly passionate about art, design, typography, astronomy, and psychology.

Eva is a late-diagnosed autistic (age 25) and a trans woman; although she has known she was trans since she was a teenager, she finally found the courage to transition in late 2021, and has lived as her authentic self ever since.

Kendall Jones

A late-diagnosed (58) male with ADHD

A career musician, Kendall studied jazz composition and arranging at Berklee College of Music in Boston, Massachusetts. He further honed his skills in composition and orchestration at UCLA (University of California Los Angeles). He is a freelance session guitarist and teacher of classical guitar.

With over 35 years of experience, Kendall specializes in electronic music and music production. His work in sound and software design, mix engineering, and synthesizer programming led to collaborations with instrument manufacturers Kurzweil and Kawai. He also lends his expertise as a consultant and programmer of performance systems for touring musicians.

Outside of music, Kendall's diverse interests include photography, and his work appears in magazines and print advertising.

Kendall is an editor for Embrace Autism and was the third member of Embrace Autism.

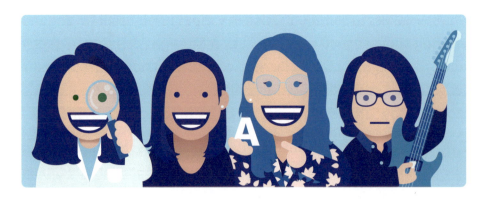

Natalie   Debra   Eva   Kendall

Acknowledgements
Nihil de nobis, sine nobis

"Nothing about us without us" (Latin: Nihil de nobis, sine nobis) is a slogan used to communicate the idea that no policy should be decided by any representative without the full and direct participation of members of the group(s) affected by that policy.

We would like to acknowledge the extraordinary debt we owe to those who contributed to this book.

Thank you to those who provided honest feedback during the creation of this book. Your feedback helped shape this book; it ensured that it was clear for medical practitioners with minimal knowledge of autism.

A special thank you to those who submitted their stories about autistic burnout (see the **Autistic Burnout Stories** section on p. 178).

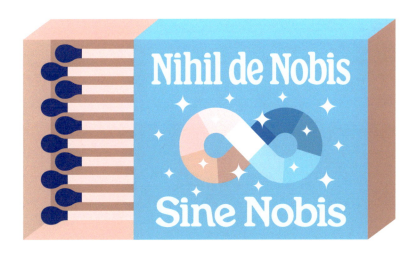

Dedication

To all adult autistics—especially those who were diagnosed later in life, and to those who feel unseen & misunderstood.

To the many respectful, trustworthy autism professionals out there who believe in patient or client-led care.

Table of Contents

Clinical Version

Non-Clinical Version

Patient Handouts

Click the link below to download a package with all the forms and other materials from the Patient Handouts section, as well as several Autistic Burnout posters you can print out:

Embrace-Autism.com/autistic-burnout-download

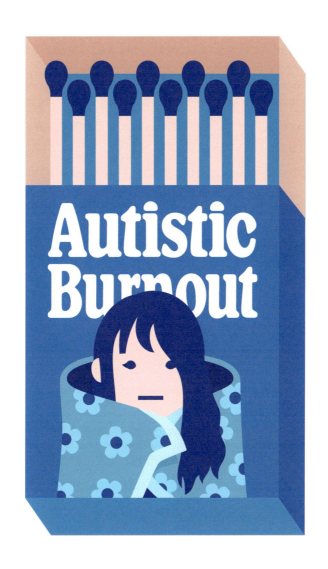

Quick Reference Guide to Autistic Burnout

Definition of Autistic Burnout

Autistic burnout is a syndrome due to chronic life stress and a mismatch of expectations and abilities without adequate support. It is characterized by pervasive, long-term (typically **3+** months) exhaustion, loss of function, and reduced tolerance to stimulus" (Raymaker et al., 2020).

Diagnostic Criteria

The provisional criteria for autistic burnout are (Higgins et al., 2021):

1. Significant mental and physical exhaustion.

2. Interpersonal withdrawal.

3. With one or more of the following factors:

- Significant reduction in social, occupational, educational, academic, behavioural, or other important areas of functioning.

- Confusion, difficulties with executive function, and dissociative states.

- Increased intensity of autistic traits and a reduced capacity to camouflage/mask autistic characteristics.

Clinical Concerns

- High risk of suicide
- Depression
- Anxiety

Screening

- Screen for suicide using the
  Ask Suicide-Screening Questionnaire (ASQ)
- ☞ www.nimh.nih.gov (search 'ASQ' in the top right, and click on the first link to the ASQ Toolkit)
- Determine the severity of autistic burnout using the **Autistic Burnout Construct** (ABO) or the **Copenhagen Burnout Inventory** (CBI)
- ☞ Embrace-Autism.com/autistic-burnout-construct
- ☞ Embrace-Autism.com/copenhagen-burnout-inventory

Treatment

- Urge the patient to take the rest they need to recover.
- Provide a medical exemption from work or school.
- Refer to an autism-focused healthcare provider equipped to assist in identifying and eliminating causal factors.
- Encourage the patient to seek support.

Defining Autistic Burnout

Autistic burnout (ABO) has been proposed as a new condition classification distinct from occupational burnout or clinical depression (Raymaker et al., 2020).

Autistic burnout results from "chronic life stress and a mismatch of expectations and abilities without adequate supports. It is characterised by pervasive, long-term (typically **3+** months) exhaustion, loss of function, and reduced tolerance to stimulus" (Raymaker et al., 2020).

In simple terms, autistic burnout is "a state of incapacitation, exhaustion, and distress in every area of life" (Raymaker et al., 2020).

The provisional criteria for autistic burnout as defined by Higgins et al. (2021) are:

1	**Significant mental and physical exhaustion**
2	**Interpersonal withdrawal**
3	**One or more of the following factors:**
A	Significant reduction in social, occupational, educational, academic, behavioural, or other important areas of functioning.
B	Confusion, difficulties with executive function, and dissociative states.
C	Increased intensity of autistic traits, and a reduced capacity to camouflage/mask autistic characteristics.

In brief, autistic burnout can look like:

1. **Feeling more emotional** than usual (e.g., easily overwhelmed, more meltdowns/shutdowns).

2. **Changes in executive functioning** (e.g., harder to plan things, more difficulty coping with unexpected changes and disruptions in routine, more difficulty making decisions).

3. **Feeling more exhausted than usual**—both physically and mentally (e.g., unable to think clearly, not being able to concentrate, having a harder time to complete work, more difficulty to remember things, need for rest, unable to keep up with social demands, etc.).

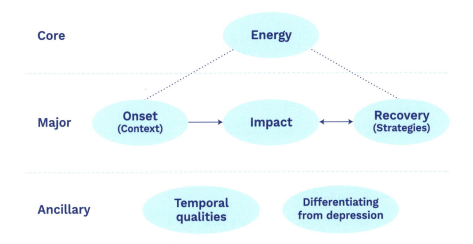

Integrative diagram and conceptual framework of autistic burnout.   Higgins et al., (2021)

The core feature of autistic burnout is (lack of) energy; major attributes are its causes, impacts, and recovery. Ancillary attributes are the duration of autistic burnout, and how it differs from depression.

Epidemiology

Prevalence of Autistic Burnout

Data published by Mantzalas et al. (2024) indicate that the prevalence of autistic burnout is **69%**, with a high rate of recurrence. It is estimated that **46%** of autistics have experienced autistic burnout four or more times in their lifetime.

Notably, a later diagnosis of autism increases the risk of experiencing autistic burnout (Matzalas et al., 2022).

Gender and racial diagnostic disparities around autistic burnout are currently unknown.

Prevalence of Autism

National Estimates

Based on estimates from the CDC's Autism and Developmental Disabilities Monitoring Network (ADDM; 2023), about **1** in **36** children age 8 are autistic (or **2.76%**; Maenner et al., 2023). This is based on data from the US; the prevalence varies per country based on differences in diagnostic rates, data collection, research methodology, and possibly racial differences as well (Zeidan et al. (2022).

Global Estimates

A systematic review update by Zeidan et al. (2022) on the global prevalence based on data from 2012 to 2021 indicates an estimated prevalence of **0.01–4.36%**, with a median of **1%**—showing the significant heterogeneity of reported prevalence rates depending on the country.

Gender Ratio

It is commonly believed that autism is more prevalent in males compared to females; however, research from Posserud et al. (2021) suggests that this is due to the timing of diagnoses; females tend to get diagnosed later in life. Accordingly, the difference in prevalence between males and females diminishes in adulthood.

- Male-to-female ratio for autistic children 4–10 years: **4.46:1**
- Male-to-female ratio for autistic children 11–17 years: **3.67:1**
- Male-to-female ratio for autistic adults 18+ years: **2.57:1**

Diagnostic Gender Bias

The male-to-female ratio of autism has shifted from **4:1** to **3:1** over the years, which shows a diagnostic gender bias (Loomes et al., 2017).

Some estimate that the true male-to-female ratio may be closer to **2:1**; but research by McCrossin (2022) using a mathematical model based on published data of autism diagnoses indicates the true ratio may even be **3:4**; they further suggest that **80%** of females remain undiagnosed at age 18.

Gender-Diverse Individuals

The prevalence rate is unclear for gender-diverse individuals; however, recent findings show that gender-diverse identities (e.g., trans, non-binary, etc) are more common in the autistic community (Warrier et al., 2020).

BIPOC Individuals

While autism occurs in all racial, ethnic, and socioeconomic groups, research shows that Black, Hispanic, and Asian autistics are more likely to be identified later in life (Aylward et al., 2021).

Interestingly, the rate of autism diagnosis for children of color has outpaced the diagnostic rate for white children. Roughly **3%** of Black, Hispanic and Asian or Pacific Islander children are diagnosed with autism, compared with about **2%** of white children (ADDM, 2023).

Risk Factors

Although burnout is caused by external factors, specific traits or characteristics can make autistic individuals more prone to experiencing autistic burnout. Such traits often lead to these individuals being more frequently exposed to chronically stressful environments and relationships where they are expected to handle demands that surpass their capabilities.

The following traits are significant risk factors for autistic burnout:

1. Low self-awareness
2. Camouflaging/masking
3. Poor mental health
4. Executive functioning challenges
5. Other factors including a history of trauma, sensory sensitivities, etc.

1. Low Self-Awareness

Low self-awareness is characterized by alexithymia and challenges with metacognition and interoception. Between **50–85%** of all autistics have co-occurring alexithymia, as opposed to just **5–13%** of the general population (Heaton et al., 2012; Kinnaird et al., 2019; Mattila et al., 2006; Salminen et al., 1999).

These individuals struggle to recognize, identify, classify, and/or describe feelings and sensations with any nuance. Many people with alexithymia are unable to differentiate between pain and fatigue or hunger and anxiety.

Furthermore, alexithymic individuals are typically only able to express affective states in general and sometimes vague categories such as sad, good, bad, and "fine".

Consequently, low self-awareness predisposes individuals to autistic burnout by:

1. Limiting one's ability to recognize stress, distress, pain, discomfort, etc.

2. Reducing one's ability to identify needs and to recognize when they are being unmet.

3. Seemingly increasing one's pain/distress tolerance because pain/distress is occurring outside of one's awareness.

4. Underreporting experiences of pain or distress due to low awareness of the actual extent, or an inability to describe them comprehensively (e.g., using vague descriptions that aren't taken seriously).

5. Misclassifying negative experiences as neutral or even positive ones.

2. Camouflaging/Masking

Camouflaging describes how some autistic individuals adopt a set of actions and strategies—consisting of compensation, masking, and assimilation—to navigate the neurotypical social world, to fit in, to cultivate connections, to prevent rejection and social ostracization, or to gain acceptance from others (Hull et al., 2017; 2018). Camouflaging demands a lot of energy and has been linked to burnout, depression, and anxiety in autistic individuals (Alaghband-rad et al., 2023).

According to the social camouflaging model (Hull et al., 2018), autistic individuals engage in three forms of camouflaging:

1. **Compensation:** Strategies used to actively compensate for difficulties in social situations (e.g., copying body language and facial expressions; learning social cues from movies and books; using pre-planned social scripts across different contexts).

2. **Masking:** Strategies used to hide autistic characteristics or portray a non-autistic persona (e.g., adjusting face and body to appear confident and/or relaxed; forcing eye contact).

3. **Assimilation:** Strategies used to try to fit in with others in social situations (e.g., putting on an act; avoiding or forcing interactions with others; feigning interest; exaggerating expressions and excitement for other people's benefit).

> ### Note
> Colloquially, masking is often used synonymously with camouflaging. However, from a clinical perspective, masking is considered a subset of camouflaging (Hull et al., 2018).

Engaging in camouflaging demands time, effort, and energy (e.g., autistic individuals have to set aside time to rehearse social interactions; acting and suppressing one's true behaviours requires more effort/energy than being authentic). This negatively impacts overall mental health (Alaghband-Rad et al., 2023; Cook et al., 2021)—further increasing the risk of experiencing/exacerbating autistic burnout.

Livingston et al. (2019) also report that autistic people who camouflage their autistic traits are often disbelieved when they disclose their autism, and are thus poorly supported because of their neurotypical presentation. This lack of support meant that exhaustion and burnout was frequent.

3. Poor Mental Health

Individuals who already struggle with mental health are more likely to experience burnout due to a reduced capacity for dealing with life stressors. In particular, autistics experience anxiety, depression, PTSD, and sleep disturbances at significantly higher rates than the general population (Morgan et al., 2020; Nimmo-Smith et al., 2019; Rumball et al., 2020).

1. **Anxiety:** The lifetime prevalence for clinical levels of anxiety in autistic individuals is between **27–79%** (Hollocks et al., 2018; Kent & Simonoff, 2017; Vasa et al., 2020); anxiety disorders are diagnosed in **20%** of autistic adults compared to just **8.7%** of non-autistics (Nimmo-Smith et al., 2019).
   → Anxiety in autistic people is further compounded by alexithymia; higher levels of alexithymia traits are associated with higher levels of anxiety traits (Milosavljevic et al., 2015).

2. **Depression:** Autistics have a **37–48.6%** lifetime prevalence rate of depression, with **25.9%** of autistics currently experiencing depression—compared to just **5%** in the general population (Hollocks et al., 2018; Hudson et al., 2019; World Health Organization, 2023).

    → Up to **83.3%** of autistic children and adolescents experience depression (Stewart et al., 2021).

3. **PTSD:** Between **44–60%** of autistic adults meet the criteria for PTSD at some point in their lifetime (Reuben et al., 2021; Rumball et al., 2020), compared to an estimated **5.6%** in the general population (Frans et al., 2005).

4. **Sleep disturbances: 64.7–73%** of autistics experience significantly more sleep difficulties—taking longer to fall asleep, experiencing more fragmented sleep, and waking up more in the middle of the night (Morgan et al., 2020).

    → Poor sleep is associated with a lower quality of life, impacting autistic individuals' ability to function day-to-day (Deserno et al., 2019).

5. **Other psychiatric conditions:** Autistic people are more likely to experience psychiatric conditions overall compared to non-autistics. For instance, nearly **70%** of autistic children and adolescents experience at least one co-occurring psychiatric condition, and nearly **40%** experience two or more (Hossain et al., 2020; DeFilippis, 2018). Co-occurring psychiatric conditions often compound the aforementioned mental health factors.

4. Executive Functioning Challenges

The majority of autistic individuals experience executive functioning challenges (Demetriou et al., 2019). Autistic individuals who struggle with aspects of executive functioning are less resilient to burnout due to reduced ability to cope with life/neurotypical circumstances.

For instance, individuals with low behavioural flexibility have difficulty with change—making coping with daily stressors more difficult. In addition, executive functioning challenges more generally lead to difficulties with managing time, completing tasks, or making seemingly simple tasks feel impossible.

These executive challenges and their impact on autistic burnout can be further exacerbated by co-occurring ADHD—another condition characterized by differences in executive functioning. Research shows that approximately **50–70%** of autistic people have co-occurring ADHD (Eaton et al., 2023).

5. Other

Other risk factors identified in the literature are those that increase an autistic individual's likelihood of developing or exacerbating burnout due to their associations with reduced capacity for managing demands and with negatively impacting mental health.

A non-exhaustive list of such factors include:

1. **A higher overall appraisal of autistic traits (Mantzalas et al., 2022)**
   → More autistic traits are generally associated with a higher difficulty in meeting the demands of neurotypical society.

2. **Sensory sensitivities (hyper/hypo)**
   → Sensory sensitivities reduce overall capacity to manage life demands due to a need to constantly expend energy managing sensory overload (Higgins et al., 2021; Mantzalas et al., 2022; Raymaker et al., 2022).

3. **A history of bullying, rejection, and trauma**
   - ⇢ Autistics experience bullying and trauma at higher rates than non-autistics. These experiences are associated with poorer mental health (Rai et al., 2018; Roberts et al., 2015).

4. **Low cognitive empathy**
   - ⇢ Defined as the ability to make inferences about others' beliefs and knowledge, low cognitive empathy is associated with reduced overall well-being (Bos & Stokes, 2019).

5. **Propensity for people-pleasing**
   - ⇢ This behaviour demands energy and effort. It is an example of camouflaging and should be interpreted as a 'fawn' trauma response; autistics may engage in it to self-protect from victimization (Pearson et al., 2022).

6. **Proneness to shame, self-judgment, and low self-worth**
   - ⇢ Autistics have an increased tendency to perceive themselves negatively due to experiences of social communication difficulties and discrimination. These factors impact overall mental health and perceived self-efficacy (Cooper et al., 2017; Nguyen et al., 2020).

Protective Factors

Autistics are at lower risk of experiencing burnout when they live authentically and have their support needs met. This requires individuals to embrace their autistic traits and learn to identify and meet their support needs.

Accordingly, protective factors include (Higgins et al., 2021; Mantzalas et al., 2021; 2022; Raymaker, 2020):

1. **'Stimming'** (i.e. fidgeting, rocking, spinning, rubbing fabric, or other self-stimulatory behaviours).
2. **'Special interests'** (i.e., engaging deeply in passions and interests).
3. **Self-awareness** (e.g., interoception, recognition of triggers).
4. **Self-efficacy** (e.g., self-care, boundary-setting).
5. **Social support** (e.g., family, friends, autistic community).
6. **Access to accommodations** and neurodivergent-affirming healthcare.

Special Cases

In this section, we reinterpret the aforementioned factors related to autistic burnout through the lens of several vulnerable populations.

1. Children and Teenagers

Parents, clinicians, and teachers must remain vigilant in monitoring signs of burnout; autistic children and teenagers tend to be more self-directed and are less likely than their neurotypical peers to seek help independently (Hosozawa et al., 2023).

They may additionally struggle with self-awareness and alexithymia—thus limiting their ability to recognize a need for support.

Autistic burnout can present when children/teenagers:

1. Spend numerous years in school masking/camouflaging.

2. Attend school five days a week.

3. Must endure sensory and social challenges at school and in extracurricular activities.

4. Attend mainstream schools where accessibility, inclusion, and accommodations tend to be lower.

5. Experience changes during puberty.

2. Young Adults

Autistic burnout contributes to university dropout and periods of unemployment in young adults. This can set back autistic individuals compared to their peers in terms of job prospects, finances, etc.

Recognizing situations where young adults are at increased risk of experiencing autistic burnout is important for identifying and setting up sustainable support systems and accommodations for the years to come.

Some unique examples of high-risk situations in young adults are:

1. Spending several years in college or work camouflaging.

2. Attending college or working full-time.

3. Absent/insufficient academic/workplace accommodations.

4. Enduring new sensory and social challenges at college or in the workforce.

5. Moving away from home for the first time.

6. Managing daily tasks alone or with a partner for the first time.

7. Living with unsupportive roommates in college dorms.

3. Periods of Significant Hormonal Fluctuations in Adulthood

Perimenopausal Adults

Hormonal fluctuations leave perimenopausal adults at an increased risk of experiencing burnout due to global impacts on cognition and mental health (Hogervorst et al., 2021).

This can be due to:

1. Behavioural inflexibility.
2. Unpredictability of mood, behaviour, and physiological changes.
3. Significant and/or novel changes in mood, behaviour, and physiology.
4. Hormonal changes impacting mental health including depression and anxiety.

Postpartum Individuals

Similar to the perimenopausal period, postpartum individuals are at increased risk of experiencing burnout due to changes to mood and executive functioning. Additionally, the significant life change associated with having to care for a new child causes significant and overwhelming disruptions in routine.

Etiology

Autistic burnout largely results from being autistic in a non-autistic world. A lack of autism awareness, a lack of social connection, social expectations and demands, and camouflaging result in an accumulation of life stressors.

Autistic burnout appears to be related to the stress experienced by autistic people in their daily lives. What is considered a significant life stressor for autistic individuals differs greatly from what is considered a significant life stressor for neurotypical individuals.

When chronic life stress and a mismatch of expectations and abilities occurs, autistic burnout can result.

In many contexts, autistic individuals have demands placed on them that would generally have little to no effect on non-autistic individuals. These include imposed social interactions, forced endurance of distressing sensory stimuli, and—more generally—environments that expect them to function similarly to neurotypicals.

Many of these demands exceed what autistic individuals can comfortably do without experiencing negative consequences. When autistics are subject to environments that force them to keep meeting (or attempting to meet) these demands, autistic burnout ensues.

Therefore, we can say that—due to the demands of living in a neurotypical-dominant society—autistic burnout arises as a result of a mismatch between expected functioning/behaviour and actual capabilities (Raymaker et al., 2020).

The following environmental factors can lead to the onset of autistic burnout:

1. Social demands
2. Sensory demands
3. Cognitive demands
4. Daily life demands
5. Insufficient support
6. Workplace discrimination

1. Social Demands

Autistic can experience burnout due to pressure from social expectations—particularly those based on neurotypical social norms.

For example:

1. **Social events:** Autistics expend significant amounts of energy attending social events such as weddings, funerals, graduations, school plays, baby showers, etc. When there isn't enough time to recover in between multiple events, this can push an individual towards burnout.

2. **Cross-neurotype communication:** The concept of Double Empathy (Milton et al., 2022) highlights the mutual difficulty for both autistics and neurotypicals to understand each other. When one's communication is perpetually misunderstood across relationships (e.g., parents, bosses, teachers, doctors, peers, colleagues), this can lead to experiences of alterity. Accordingly, being in environments where cross-neurotype communication is common can lead to burnout.

2. Sensory Demands

Continued unmet sensory needs—such as exposure to fluorescent lights, perfume odours, background noise, etc.—lead to prolonged stress/pain, and impede overall functioning, resulting in burnout (de Vries, 2021). Many autistics are hypersensitive to sensory stimuli; **>96%** experience sensory processing disorders (Marco et al., 2011). In sensory processing disorder, what are typically considered neutral or pleasant sensory stimuli can be extremely distressing and painful.

3. Cognitive Demands

Significant or continuous change can cause burnout. Autistics commonly struggle with behavioural flexibility (D'Cruz et al., 2013). As such, autistics tend to prefer/require sameness, routine, rituals, and predictable patterns of behaviour to manage stress. Notably, these changes do not necessarily have to be negative to cause distress and/or burnout. It is the change itself—not the outcome nor the events mediating the change—that causes overwhelm and eventually leads to autistic burnout.

For example:

1. 'Small' changes in routine: needing to take a different route; having to eat a different meal; being unexpectedly greeted by someone; receiving a negative review at work; wearing a different pair of shoes; cancelling/rescheduling plans; misplacing an item.

2. 'Large' changes in routine: starting/leaving a job; beginning a new semester at school; moving to a new home; getting a pet; losing an item of significant value; transitioning from high school to university; welcoming a newborn into the family.

3. Changes in relationships: starting to date someone; making a new friend; experiencing a break-up; getting a new boss; grieving the loss of a person.

> **Note**
>
> The magnitude of changes are subjective. While this list provides common examples, it is not comprehensive; and it does not represent how all autistic individuals appraise the changes they experience.

4. Daily Life Demands

Managing daily tasks can take a significant toll, and may eventually lead to autistic burnout. The combination of executive challenges, social and sensory differences, tasks that are often considered "errands" or weekly "to-dos" by neurotypicals, etc., demand a lot of effort and energy for autistic individuals. The dynamic interplay of responsibilities, organization, and social interactions can cause enormous cognitive load and takes strenuous effort to maintain.

For example:

1. Going to the grocery store or other shopping experiences.
2. Paying bills or doing taxes.
3. Filling in forms or other administrative work.
4. Navigating public transit, driving, or reading maps.
5. Ordering food at a restaurant or knowing how to leave a restaurant at the end of a meal.
6. Going to medical appointments or getting haircuts.
7. Cooking meals that require multiple simultaneous steps, a variety of ingredients, cooking methods/times, etc.

> **Note**
>
> It is important to be mindful that while many neurotypicals may consider some of these daily tasks to be annoying, boring, tiring, etc., for autistics, these tasks are overwhelming and exhausting.

5. Insufficient Support

Autistic individuals who experience burnout generally do not have sufficient supports in place. This refers to experiencing a lack of inclusion, support networks, accessibility, and accommodations. Autism is classified as a developmental disability (Centers for Disease Control and Prevention, 2022), implying that autistic individuals benefit from ongoing supports to varying degrees.

However, it is difficult to access sufficient levels of support while living in a neurotypical-dominant world that isn't accommodating to the needs of autistic people. An overall lack of autism awareness and accommodations at school, home, or work results in constant demands of autistic individuals which exceed their capacity (Mantzalas et al., 2022).

Here are some consequences of insufficient support for the well-being of autistics and how these experiences contribute to and/or exacerbate burnout:

1. Not being believed when you disclose that you need help.

2. Invalidation and not feeling seen or heard (e.g., being labelled 'lazy' instead of being met with compassion and support).

3. Lack of social connection and belonging; experiences of loneliness—which causes greater distress in autistic people than in neurotypicals (Quadt et al., 2023).

4. Exhaustion and energy depletion.

5. Added cognitive and emotional load.

6. Low self-worth and feeling 'less than'.

7. Self-criticism and a lack of self-compassion; feeling you're not capable enough but telling yourself you "should" be able to.

8. Comparing your experiences to those of non-autistics; holding yourself to the same expectations.

9. Negative evaluation and social rejection; judgements by others.

10. Lack of autism awareness at schools, home, or work (Attwood and Garnett, 2024; Autistic Burnout Seminar).

6. Workplace Discrimination

Autistics experience high levels of workplace discrimination (Cooper & Mujtaba, 2022). Discrimination can be direct, such as explicit ableist comments and denying accommodations; or indirect such as getting passed for a promotion or an employment opportunity without justification (Ontario Human Rights Commission, n.d.). Findings show that applicants who disclose their disability such as autism received **26%** fewer expressions of employer interest (Ameri et al., 2017).

Anecdotally, unintentional discrimination against autistics can take the form of employers altering working conditions, making it harder for autistic individuals to cope (e.g., removing hybrid work options).

Additionally, work colleagues can have distant, exclusionary, and discriminatory attitudes (Lindsay & Cancelliere, 2017; Fichten et al., 2005). These factors—especially in combination with a lack of autism awareness and appropriate accommodations—eventually result in burnout and resignation for many autistic people.

Clinical Approach

When working with individuals with autistic burnout, the following flowchart outlines the optimal course of action:

1. Screen for suicide risk

2. Diagnose and determine cause and severity of autistic burnout

    a. Conduct a clinical interview

        i. Collect a thorough history

        ii. Assess for environmental factors

        iii. Assess for risk factors

    b. Administer psychometrics

    c. Diagnose based on the current understanding of diagnostic criteria

3. Treat autistic burnout

    a. Achieve remission of autistic burnout symptoms

    b. Restore optimal functioning

    c. Prevent relapse/recurrence

A Note About Working with Autistic Individuals in Clinical Practice

Autistic individuals have different communication needs than non-autistics. Clinicians should follow these basic guidelines when meeting with autistics:

1. **Avoid social chitchat.** This is unnecessary for building rapport; and more often than not, it causes distress, anxiety, and overwhelm.

2. **Avoid assumptions based on nonverbal cues.** Autistic body language is unconventional compared to non-autistic communication norms, and should not be used as a means to gather information.

→ **Examples of typical nonverbal communication styles in autistic individuals:**

    a. "Unusual" or absent eye contact

    b. Less emotive facial expressions

    c. Less variations in tone of voice

3. **Avoid conflations between response styles and disinterest/resistance.** Autistic individuals often do not follow expected social norms in communication. Take the content of what is being said at face value and ask for clarity if there is uncertainty. For instance, sounding aloof does not signify disinterest or lack of motivation.

4. **Communicate with clarity.** Autistic individuals are typically very literal. It is necessary to communicate directly (this is not "rude" or "insensitive"!) and avoid ambiguities, implied meanings, and spaces to "fill in the blanks." Clear communication can be facilitated by:

    a. Asking specific instead of open-ended questions.

    b. Asking directly about the topic you are interested in. You cannot expect autistics to "know where you are going" with your inquiries.

    c. Explaining the purpose of your inquiry before asking a question instead of assuming you are both on the same page.

5. **Give time for responses.** Autistics may take more time than non-autistics to process questions and generate responses. To ensure you are gathering accurate information, autistics should not feel pressured to respond immediately.

→ This can be facilitated by:

    a. Sharing questions/discussion topics ahead of your meeting.

    b. Allowing individuals to follow up with more information after the meeting.

6. **Ask about communication needs.** Meet autistic individuals with dignity and agency by asking them about their needs.

→ For example:

    a. "Is there anything about the way you communicate that would be helpful for me to understand?"

    b. "Is there anything that you need from me to facilitate communication between us?"

These guidelines were developed based on the lived experiences of writers and the **Wales Autism Research Centre** (WARC) at Cardiff University (Winn, 2015).

Note

Every autistic will differ in their communication needs. The best practice is to ask about theirs!

---

1. Screen for Suicide Risk

It is imperative that clinicians begin by assessing suicide risk. Suicidality is extremely high in autistics. Up to **72%** of autistics report suicidal ideation, and up to **47%** report attempting suicide (Newell et al., 2023). Autistics are **25** times more likely to attempt suicide compared to non-autistics (Conner, 2023).

Before proceeding with the burnout assessment, administer the **Ask Suicide-Screening Questionnaire** (ASQ)—an evidence-based suicide screening tool developed by the National Institute of Mental Health (Horowitz et al., 2020). It generally takes about **1** minute to administer.

Ask your patient the following:

1. In the past few weeks, have you wished you were dead?　　　　　　　　　　　　○ Yes　○ No
2. In the past few weeks, have you felt that you or your family would be better off if you were dead?　○ Yes　○ No
3. In the past week, have you been having thoughts about killing yourself?　　　　　○ Yes　○ No
4. Have you ever tried to kill yourself?　　　○ Yes　○ No
    → If yes, how? _____
    → When? _____

If the patient answers 'Yes' to any of the above, ask the following acuity question:

5. Are you currently having thoughts of killing yourself?　　　　　　　　　　　　　○ Yes　○ No
    → If yes, please describe: _____

Next steps:

- If patient answers 'No' to all questions 1 through 4, screening is complete (not necessary to ask question #5). No intervention is necessary.

- If patient answers 'Yes' to any of questions 1 through 4, or refuses to answer, they are considered a positive screen.

> ### Note
> Clinical judgment can always override a negative screen.

- 'Yes' to question #5 = **acute positive screen** (imminent risk identified).
  - → Patient requires a **STAT** safety/full mental health evaluation.
  - → Patient cannot leave until evaluated for safety.
- 'No' to question #5 = **non-acute positive screen** (potential risk identified).
  - → Patient requires a brief suicide safety assessment to determine if a full mental health evaluation is needed. If a patient (or parent/guardian) refuses the brief assessment, this should be treated as an 'against medical advice' (AMA) discharge.
  - → Alert the physician or clinician responsible for the patient's care.

The provider must first assess suicidality and then determine why the person is experiencing it. The ASK suicide protocol should be followed.

When the Patient is Suicidal

If a person is suicidal, a screener for autistic burnout should still be done so that the patient has the relevant information they require. Ideally, we want to ensure that this person is referred to someone specialized in autism who knows what to do.

However, if the patient must go to the hospital, it is essential that they are provided with a handout for practitioners, such as our **Quick Reference Guide to Autistic Burnout** at the start of this book—in addition to a note explaining that they are autistic and have been assessed for autistic burnout.

2. Diagnose and Determine the Severity of Autistic Burnout

The basis for an autistic burnout diagnosis depends on:

1. The individual being autistic.
2. Significant mental and physical exhaustion and interpersonal withdrawal.
3. A reduction in overall functioning, executive functioning, and ability to hide autistic traits.

To comprehensively understand the individual's condition, clinicians should conduct a clinical interview, administer psychometrics, and compare their presentation with the diagnostic criteria.

> ### Note
> There are currently no objective tests that unequivocally diagnose autistic burnout.

Clinical Interview

Interview the individual to identify:

1. **The nature and duration of autistic burnout symptoms.**

    → A thorough history is required to identify the external factors causing autistic burnout and maintaining autistic burnout. Determining risk factors facilitating autistic burnout is necessary ahead of treatment.

    → A comprehensive list of causes of autistic burnout and risk factors can be found in the **Etiology** section (p. 40) of this guidebook.

2. **The age of onset.**

3. **Any previous episodes of autistic burnout.**

4. **The impact of symptoms on functioning.**

    → **The Signs of Autistic Burnout** section (p. 70) of this guidebook characterizes the scope of burnout symptoms and impacts on functioning.

5. **Rule out or diagnose potentially co-occurring conditions such as depression, anxiety disorders, PTSD, and occupational burnout.**

    → Refer to the **Differential Diagnoses** section (p. 72) of this guidebook.

6. **Rule out physical causes.**

    → For example, long COVID, cardiovascular disease, thyroid conditions, chronic fatigue, dysautonomia, and Postural Orthostatic Tachycardia Syndrome (POTS) are common concurrences with autism.

> **Note**
>
> Due to the high degree of overlap and misdiagnosis of depression and autistic burnout, autistic individuals who present with depression or suicidality should be screened for autistic burnout.

On the following pages you can find different psychometrics you can use to assess for autistic burnout, followed by a listing of provisional criteria for autistic burnout.

Psychometrics

The following screening/assessment tools are recommended for use by primary healthcare professionals when autistic burnout is suspected:

Psychometrics for Autistic Burnout

Autistic Burnout Construct (ABO; Richards et al., 2023): this self-assessment tool consists of 8 questions measuring the *Exhaustion* dimension of autistic burnout. It has demonstrated strong psychometric properties, including internal consistency, and convergent and divergent validity. You can find an automated version at Embrace-Autism.com > Autism tests > Other tests.

Copenhagen Burnout Inventory (CBI; Kristensen et al., 2005): this self-report measure consists of 19 items, which measures three types of burnout: personal burnout, work-related burnout, and client-related burnout. All three scales were found to have very high internal reliability. The *Personal Burnout* subscale was found to correlate with autistic burnout (Mantzalas et al., 2024). As such, use the 8-item CBI–P to measure autistic burnout specifically.

However, we found it useful to take the complete CBI to get a sense of what aspects contribute most significantly to burnout in general; the demands imposed by the latter two domains will have an impact on autistic burnout as well.

Psychometrics for Autism

Embrace autism has a wide range of automated psychometric tests to screen for autism. See the list of psychometrics at our tests page:

Embrace-Autism.com/autism-tests

Ritvo Autism Asperger Diagnostic Scale–Revised (RAADS–R; Ritvo et al., 2010): administration of this sensitive and specific questionnaire is recommended to identify adult autistics who "escape diagnosis" due to a subclinical level presentation.

The Autism Spectrum Quotient (AQ; Baron-Cohen, 2001): a self-administered questionnaire used to measure autistic traits in adults (age 16+). An IQ of at least low average (IQ >=80) is required to take the test adequately.

> **Note**
>
> Some of the items on the AQ are outdated (read the **Updated** section of our Embrace Autism article on the AQ for suggestions on a more contemporary/generalized interpretation of these items.

Psychometrics for Depression

Beck Depression Inventory-II (BD-II; Beck et al., 1996): administration of the BDI-II (or another screening tool for depression) is recommended considering **98%** of individuals with autistic burnout meet the threshold for a diagnosis of depression (Arnold et al., 2023; Mantzalas, 2024).

Psychometrics for Occupational Burnout

Copenhagen Burnout Inventory (CBI; Kristensen et al., 2005): this self-assessment tool measures three types of burnout: personal burnout, work-related burnout, and client-related burnout. All three scales were found to have very high internal reliability. Use the *Work-related Burnout* subscale to measure occupational burnout specifically.

Maslach Burnout Inventory™ (MBI; Masclack et al., 1996): this tool allows clinicians to screen for occupational burnout; this may be present alongside autistic burnout, and may exacerbate it.

Diagnostic Criteria

Despite burnout being first identified in 1974 (Freudenberger, 1974), the World Health Organization (WHO) is the only significant health organization to legitimize burnout with its inclusion in the 11th Edition of the International Classification of Diseases (ICD-11; WHO, 2019).

The American Psychiatric Association (APA) has yet to consider autistic burnout—as well as occupational burnout—a recognized condition in the DSM-5-TR (American Psychiatric Association, 2022).

However, its working group on well-being and burnout is taking the topic seriously, and has even offered its members a way to evaluate their own burnout. Until the APA has released official diagnostic criteria, researchers have developed provisional criteria for autistic burnout (Higgins et al., 2021).

The provisional criteria for autistic burnout, according to Higgins et al. (2021), are:

The following symptoms must have been present for a period of at least **3** months, and represent a change from previous functioning:

1. **Significant mental and physical exhaustion—often described as extreme fatigue.** This profound exhaustion, the central feature of autistic burnout, is an overwhelming sense of exhaustion. It goes beyond ordinary tiredness and significantly impacts an individual's physical and emotional well-being.

2. **Interpersonal withdrawal, resulting in reduced social engagement.** Burnout often leads to increased social withdrawal. Autistic individuals may find it challenging to engage in social interactions during this period, opting for solitude as a means of coping.

3. **One or more of the following:**
   a. Significant reduction in functioning in various areas (e.g., social, occupational, educational).
   b. Confusion, difficulties with executive function, and/or dissociative states.
   c. Increased intensity of autistic traits and/or reduced capacity to camouflage/mask autistic characteristics and/or reduced tolerance of stimuli.

Note

Autistic burnout is not better explained by a psychiatric illness such as depression, psychosis, personality disorders, or trauma- and stressor-related disorders.

Caveats

There are a few things to keep in mind when diagnosing autistic burnout (Higgins et al., 2021):

1. Extended or chronic episodes of autistic burnout may be preceded by brief or intermittent episodes.
2. It can be difficult to identify the extent of burnout, as the person may have brief energy bursts—usually related to positive stimulation—though overall be debilitated.
3. Burnout has an appearance of an inbuilt survival mechanism.

Diagnostic Criteria for Autistic Burnout

Autistic burnout is characterized by:

① Significant Exhaustion

② Increased Social Withdrawal

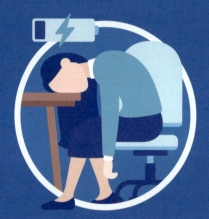 +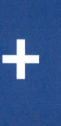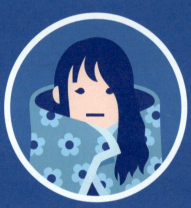

③ Plus one or more of the following:

Ⓐ Reduction in Functioning

Ⓑ More Executive Challenges

Ⓒ Reduced Capacity to Camouflage

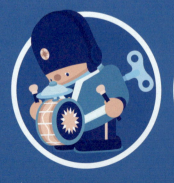 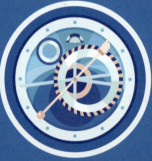 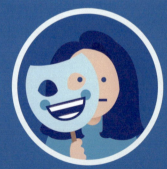

Provisional criteria for autistic burnout according to Higgins et al. (2021).

Autistic burnout can look like:

Greater Emotionality

→ Feeling more emotional
→ Prone to getting overwhelmed
→ Difficulty regulating emotions
→ Experiencing more meltdowns
→ Experiencing more shutdowns

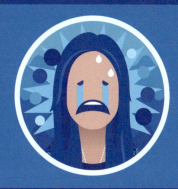

Executive Challenges

→ More difficulty planning things
→ More difficulty coping with unexpected changes
→ More difficulty coping with disruptions in routine
→ More difficulty making decisions

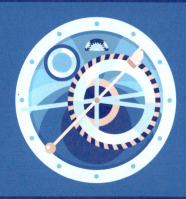

Significant Exhaustion

→ Feeling physically more exhausted
→ Feeling mentally more exhausted
→ Unable to think clearly
→ Difficulty concentrating
→ A harder time completing work
→ Difficulty remembering things
→ More need for rest
→ Unable to keep up with social demands

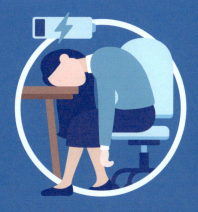

Common symptoms of autistic burnout according to Higgins et al. (2021).

3. Treating Autistic Burnout

In this section, we share an autistic-affirming treatment protocol for autistic burnout.

Treatment recommendations are based on research as well as the lived experiences of autistic individuals (Mantzalas et al., 2022; Raymaker et al., 2020).

Treatment Protocol

Preliminary: Assess for Suicide Risk

Step 1: Identify

1. Have the patient fill out the **Energy Inventory** (p. 220) from the **Patient Handouts** section (p. 216)

> ### Note
> Filling in this form may be difficult for autistics with low self-awareness, alexithymia, and challenges with interoception. Accordingly, individuals may require support to facilitate recognition.

2. Interview the patient to identify high demand life situations (a comprehensive list of relevant factors for assessment can be found in the **Etiology** section; p. 40):
   a. **Demands:** social demands, sensory demands, cognitive demands, daily life demands
   b. **Change:** life transitions
   c. **Parenting and relationships:** single parent, conflict in child-rearing styles, mismatch in neurotype (i.e., one person is autistic and the other is neurotypical)

d. **Employment:** full-time work, in-person work, amount of social interaction at work, autism awareness at work, commute

   e. **School:** lack of accommodations, full-time

   f. **Co-occurrences:** ADHD, MCAS, POTS

Step 2: Retreat

1. Medical leave

   a. Duration is dependent on severity and length of autistic burnout

   b. Reassess autistic burnout score using the **Autistic Burnout Construct** (ABO) and/or the **Copenhagen Burnout Inventory** (CBI) every **2** months

2. Accommodation letter

   a. Part-time hours

   b. Work from home

   c. Sensory accommodation

3. Withdraw from demands (use the **Energy Inventory** on p. 220 of the **Patient Handouts** section to identify things that feel too demanding/draining to the patient)

   a. Practical, realistic

   b. Suggest patient inform people that withdrawal is not personal

4. Prognosis

   a. In order to prevent severe/prolonged burnout, retreat should occur as soon as possible

   b. Recovering from burnout can take months or years if the level of burnout is severe

Step 3: Restructure

1. Environmental modification is necessary; autistic burnout is an environmental problem, not an autistic person problem.

2. Suggest the patient consult an experienced autistic therapist who is knowledgeable about autistic burnout to find ways to avoid or accommodate high levels of stress.

3. Have the patient consider seeking disability leave for a period of time in order to recuperate.

4. Help the patient accept that, to prevent autistic burnout re-occurrence, they cannot return to what caused the burnout (e.g., your job, your relationship).

5. Identify support needs and establish accommodations and social supports.

Seek support:

1. **Help the patient consider ways to communicate their needs to others.**
   a. Explain their daily challenges using speech, text, email, etc.
   b. Ask for help from friends and loved ones.
   c. If safe, speak to human resources at work, a disability coordinator at school, and seek out a primary care physician, therapist, etc.

2. **Connect with others in the autistic community**
   a. Join a social support network online.
   b. Look for others on social media (e.g. by searching the hashtag **#ActuallyAutistic** on Twitter/X).
   c. Seek out an autistic mentor.

Step 4: Re-energize

1. Encourage the patient to list activities that re-energizes them, and ensure that they regularly engage in them.

2. Engage in special interests during recovery (energy permitting) and create a plan for continued engagement ahead of step 5.

Step 5: Return and Reintegrate

It is advised to begin this step only once the person's score is **31** or lower on the **ABO**, and/or **49** or lower on the **CBI–P**—or if their score is significantly lower than their initial score.

Gradual return:

1. Help the patient in the following ways:
   a. Re-integrate with the external world in a graduated manner.
   b. Return to daily activities and routines at a reduced level at school or work.
   c. Start with half of what they believe they can do.

2. Monitor for signs according to **Identify** (step 1) and return to **Retreat** (step 2) at the earliest signs of burnout.

Note

Further restructuring and reconfiguring may be needed before reintegration is sustainable. Reintegration may be an iterative process of relapsing and remitting, especially if significant environmental changes and social supports are necessary. Identifying needs and accepting limitations can be difficult.

Drop the Mask

Given that masking/camouflaging is a significant risk factor for autistic burnout due to energy and emotional demands, being more selective about when to engage in this coping mechanism is crucial for recovery and prevention.

1. In situations where individuals are accustomed to automatically masking/camouflaging, promote more deliberate choices that encourage these strategies when it is more beneficial than harmful.

2. Prioritize authenticity.

Note

Masking and camouflaging can be ways for autistics to stay safe and self-protect in discriminatory and exclusionary environments—particularly for autistics who hold multiple marginalized identities (e.g., queer, trans, and BIPOC autistics). It may not be safe or realistic for an autistic individual to completely unmask in all situations. A more realistic goal may be 'masking in moderation' rather than completely unmasking.

Importantly, the relationship between safety/self-protection and masking applies to the therapeutic relationship. Clinicians working with autistic individuals must cultivate a safe and inclusive environment for autistics. Camouflaging is a significant barrier to receiving support.

Conventional Psychotherapy Approaches

When dealing with autistic burnout, the general advice is for individuals to seek counselling/psychotherapy. However, autistic burnout is not included in clinical training programs, so expertise is lacking.

It is crucial that clinicians understand that autistic burnout is an environmental problem—not an individual, personal, or character flaw. Rather, autistic burnout should be considered an adaptive response to an environment that does not suit that person.

As outlined above, treatment approaches should focus on:

1. Withdrawing from demands to facilitate recovery.
2. Identifying precipitating and perpetuating environmental factors.
3. Identifying predisposing situations and traits.
4. Identifying individual support needs.

In contrast, conventional psychotherapies typically aim to shift a person's patterns of thought and behaviour instead of addressing environmental factors (e.g., in CBT, ACT, and DBT). Conventional psychotherapies should therefore be used with caution. Cognitive restructuring techniques and appraising autistic traits as maladaptive or impaired is not a neurodivergent-affirming approach to counselling (Chapman & Botha, 2023).

Here are some ways that conventional psychotherapy is contraindicated for autistic individuals:

1. **Cognitive Behaviour Therapy** that characterizes autistic burnout as a form of distorted thinking rather than a genuine need for rest and withdrawal is harmful. Further, differences in executive functioning and energy depletion are likely to adversely affect the efficacy of CBT in autistic individuals. And finally, cognitive overload has been identified as a stressor that can lead to onset of autistic burnout, and CBT could further add to the cognitive load experienced by autistic adults (Arnold et al., 2023).

2. **Talk therapy** that is unstructured and open-ended may be difficult for an autistic to navigate. Autistics may require more structured session with explicit direction.

3. **Distress tolerance techniques (e.g., DBT) and exposure therapies** exacerbate autistic burnout and cause further harm.

4. **Psychotherapy and counselling-based on neurotypical needs and behavioural norms** are considered unethical therapeutic approaches for autistic people. Autistic burnout is an adaptive response to an environment that encourages and/or forces autistic individuals to tolerate situations that are detrimental to them, so this should not be replicated in a therapeutic context (Chapman & Botha, 2023).

When is Psychotherapy/Counselling Appropriate?

Psychological therapies necessitate adaptations in order to be accessible and effective for autistic individuals. Therapists need to have an understanding of autistic traits and needs.

Most of all, assumptions should not be made based on a diagnosis of autism (Fisher et al., 2023)—psychotherapy should not aim to "decrease autism symptoms" (Chapman & Botha, 2023).

Here are some examples of adaptations/accommodations:

1. Virtual therapy is typically more comfortable and has equal efficacy for autistic adults. This reduces many barriers related to accessing healthcare such as increased comfort, eliminating the need to travel, ensuring a sensory-friendly environment, eliminating the need to interact with secretaries and crowded waiting rooms, etc. (Harris et al., 2022).

2. Removing sensory stressors such as bright lights and loud ambient noises.

3. Making appointments routine so that the date, time, and place are predictable.

4. Alter communication styles by asking more direct questions, not requiring eye-contact, using a consistent tone of voice, etc.

5. Offer accommodations to reduce uncertainty such as an agenda ahead of each session, an explanation of the activity prior to engaging experientially, etc.

With appropriate adaptations and accommodations in place, psychotherapy can be helpful for supporting autistics experiencing mental health challenges. Supporting autistic mental health is crucial for preventing autistic burnout (see **Risk Factors** at p. 30).

Pharmacological Treatments

Autistic burnout does not require pharmacological treatment, as it is caused by external factors rather than internal physiological differences.

However, medications—such as SSRIs—may help treat autistic burnout indirectly by supporting autistics who have co-occurring conditions such as depression and anxiety.

> ### Note
> Many existing studies have used medications to target core features of autism rather than targeting mental health conditions. Using medications in this way does not help autistic people (Linden et al., 2022). It serves to stigmatize and pathologize autistics. Autistic traits do not need to be "cured" or "reduced".

Co-occurrences

Autistic burnout commonly occurs alongside:

1. **Depression**
   - → Arnold et al. (2023) found that **98%** of autistics with autistic burnout meet the criteria for Major Depressive Disorder.

2. **Occupational burnout**
   - → A global survey by the McKinsey Institute (2022) featuring 15,000 employees in 15 countries found that the prevalence of occupational burnout in the general population ranged from **19–38%**, with on average 1 in 4 employees surveyed reporting experiencing burnout symptoms. These statistics apply to autistic people as well; and given that there is some overlap between occupational and autistic burnout in terms of imposed demands and lack of support to deal with those demands, autistic people may be particularly susceptible to occupational burnout.
   - → Kovács et al. (2023) cite that risk factors for occupational burnout were (**1**) being female, (**2**) having a lower quality of life, (**3**) experiencing chronic pain, (**4**) mental health struggles, and (**5**) sleep disturbance. These are common lived experiences in the autistic population (Ayres et al., 2018; Nimmo-Smith et al., 2019; Rumball et al., 2020; Whitney & Shapiro, 2019), suggesting that autistic individuals are more susceptible to occupational burnout than the general population.

3. **ADHD**
   - → Based on pooled prevalence estimates, approximately **50–70%** of autistic people have co-occurring ADHD (Eaton et al., 2023).
   - → Note that just like autistic traits, ADHD traits may become more prominent during burnout.

4. **Alexithymia**
   - → A higher prevalence of alexithymia has been reported among autistics; **49.93%** compared to **4.89%** in the general population (Kinnaird et al., 2019).
   - → The prevalence rates of alexithymia in the autism groups from Kinnaird et al. (2019) ranged from **33.3%** to **63%**, with a mean weighted prevalence rate of **49.93%**.

5. **Autoimmune conditions**
   - → Autistic people have a significantly higher prevalence of allergic and autoimmune diseases, including an increased risks of **asthma** (OR = **1.74**), **allergic rhinitis** (OR = **1.70**), **atopic dermatitis** (OR = **1.52**), **urticaria** (OR = **1.38**) and **type 1 diabetes** (OR = **4.00**), and a trend toward increasing comorbidity with **Crohn's disease** (OR = **1.46**) (M. Chen et al., 2013).
   - → Children born to mothers with autoimmune disease are **34%** more likely to be autistic (Chen et al., 2016).

6. **PTSD**
   - → Approximately **60%** of autistics reported probable PTSD in their lifetime (compare this to **4.5%** of the general population) (Rumball, 2020).

Characterizing Autistic Burnout

Autistic burnout develops as a result of chronic life stress, a mismatch between expectations and abilities, and insufficient supports. It is generally characterized by exhaustion, cognitive changes, more apparent autistic traits, and withdrawal from social interaction.

Signs of Autistic Burnout

The ECAO acronym was developed to classify signs of autistic burnout. It was created by Arnold et al. (2023) based on the **Autistic Burnout Severity Items** (ABSI).

1. **Exhaustion (E)**
   a. Exhaustion (mental and physical) and social withdrawal
   b. A desire to do as little as possible
   c. Potential worsening of physical health
      → E.g., chronic fatigue
   d. Low self-esteem and self-efficacy; former coping mechanisms are no longer helpful and previously enjoyable things no longer are
   e. Dropping out of university and/or unemployment
   f. Signs of exhaustion persist for months to years

2. **Cognitive Disruption (C), Memory Problems, Confusion, and Mood**
   a. Reduction in functioning compared to the baseline
      → E.g., reduced self-care, emotional dysregulation, selective mutism

b. New executive functioning challenges

→ E.g., it may appear as though the individual has acquired ADHD-like traits

c. Reduction in cognitive processing

→ E.g., 'brain fog'

d. Confusion as to whether the signs are indicative of clinical depression (this confusion may be experienced by the individual or by clinicians unfamiliar with autistic burnout)

e. Difficulty reporting emotional exhaustion (alexithymia) and asking for help

f. Decreased sense of personal accomplishment

g. Overall worsening of mental health and changes in mood.

→ E.g., despair, negativity, depression, irritability, suicidality

3. **Heightened Autistic Self-Awareness (A)**

a. Increased sensory sensitivity and self-awareness of autistic characteristics

b. Increased manifestation of autistic traits

→ Note: many autistic traits are considered coping mechanisms, thus this increase signifies an increase in engagement with coping techniques (e.g., increased 'stimming')

c. Decrease in camouflaging

d. Likely due to a reduced capacity to camouflage rather than a choice to reduce camouflaging behaviour

e. May precede and precipitate a diagnosis of autism

f. Reduced tolerance to sensory and social input

4. **Overwhelm and Withdrawal (O)**
   a. More shutdowns
      → E.g., being frozen (an inability to do anything—or even to move)
   b. Need for social withdrawal and recovery/downtime
   c. Can include complete social isolation
   d. Suicidal ideation, attempt, or completion
   e. Brought on by feelings of 'needing a way out'
   f. **44%** of autistics in burnout experience suicidality (Higgins et al., 2021)

> ### Note
> Shutdowns can mimic the characteristics of burnout, but shutdowns are transient and last for minutes to days; whereas burnout is chronic and lasts from months to years.

Differential Diagnoses

Autistic burnout is often mischaracterized as depression, occupational burnout, or chronic fatigue. This can delay recovery and even worsen symptoms. Therefore, familiarizing yourself with how to differentiate between these conditions is necessary when working with autistics.

Depression vs. Autistic Burnout

Roughly **98%** of autistic individuals experiencing autistic burnout exceed the cut-off for a diagnosis of depression, indicating a significant overlap (Arnold et al., 2023; Richards et al., 2023). Yet, burnout and depression have distinct etiologies and incompatible treatment approaches. Conflating autistic burnout symptoms with depression can delay recovery and cause further harm.

> ## "Depression is the side effect, with burnout being the cause"
>
> ### Participant in the research of Arnold et al. (2023)

Here is a summary of how depression and autistic burnout compare (Arnold et al., 2023; Raymaker et al., 2020):

Autistic Burnout	Depression
1. Behavioural change	
An apparent increase in autistic traits, such as sensory sensitivities, difficulty processing social and emotional information, and increased desire for repetition and sameness.	A change in mood, such as feeling low, despondent, and despair. Triad of maladaptive thinking. For example, thinking, "I am bad, the world is bad, and it is always going to be this way."
2. Passions and interests	
Engaging in 'special interests' is energizing.	Reduced enjoyment of passions and interests.
3. Social withdrawal	
Pervasive, and considered a coping mechanism; a recovery tool.	Social withdrawal can be a cause and furtherance of depression.
4. Somatic symptoms	
Increased fatigue potentially requiring more sleep to recover, but sleep disturbance is not a main feature.	Appetite and sleep disturbances; increased sleep does not promote recovery.

Occupational Burnout

Definitions of occupational burnout vary in the research literature; but according to one of the most influential approaches, burnout is conceptualised as a response to prolonged job stress characterised by three dimensions (Maslach et al., 2001):

1. Exhaustion

2. Cynicism

3. Lack of accomplishment

An autistic with occupational burnout may present with similar symptoms to someone with autistic burnout (Canadian Psychology Association, 2021).

However, unlike occupational burnout, autistic burnout has a variety of non-work-related causes. Limiting diagnoses to occupational burnout prevents autistics who are experiencing other forms of burnout from receiving the necessary support for recovery and relapse prevention.

Autistic burnout—but not occupational burnout—can be caused by:

1. Social demands

2. Sensory demands

3. Demands of daily tasks

4. Changes in routine and unexpected life events

5. Insufficient levels of support (inclusion, accessibility, accommodations)

Comparisons with Occupational Burnout

Most importantly, autistic burnout is a distinct phenomenon from occupational burnout. The conditions have unique etiologies, and an autistic can have both autistic burnout and occupational burnout (Raymaker et al., 2020).

Exhaustion is a core feature in both occupational and autistic burnout, but the etiologies are distinct. However, occupational burnout in autistic people may show some overlap with autistic burnout in terms of demands imposed on them, versus the lack of support to deal with those demands. This is exemplified in the theoretical model of resources and demands by Tomczak & Kulikowski (2023), based on the Job Demands-Resources for Autism model by Bury et al. (2022).

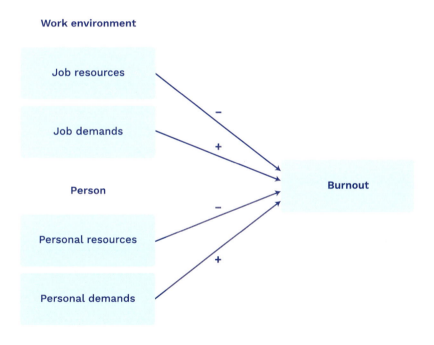

Theoretical model of resources and demands influencing burnout, constituting a framework for our conceptual analysis of burnout among employees with autism based on Job Demands-Resources Theory (Bakker & Demerouti, 2017)

Autistic individuals can experience burnout due to a host of other prolonged periods of general stress—many of which include but also go beyond the context of work relationships. Therefore, the rate of occupational burnout in the autistic population is thought to be much higher than in neurotypicals, and much higher than the **25%** cited for occupational burnout (Raymaker et al., 2020).

The prevalence rate of occupational burnout fluctuates depending on the profession and working conditions. Overall, **25%** of workers report burnout, but estimates from the last five years are as high as **50%** for postal workers (Kovács et al., 2023); **56.6%** for resident physicians (Dhusia et al., 2019); and **23.9%** for physical education teachers (Alsalhe et al., 2021).

To this point, in postal workers—where the rate of occupational burnout was much higher than average—Kovács et al. (2023) cite that risk factors for occupational burnout were (**1**) being female, (**2**) having a lower quality of life, (**3**) experiencing chronic pain, (**4**) mental health struggles, and (**5**) sleep disturbance. These are common lived experiences in the autistic population (Ayres et al., 2018; Nimmo-Smith et al., 2019; Rumball et al., 2020; Whitney & Shapiro, 2019), suggesting that autistic individuals are more susceptible to burnout than the general population.

Chronic Fatigue Syndrome

Myalgic encephalomyelitis/chronic fatigue syndrome (ME/CFS) is a chronic illness with overlapping symptoms to autistic burnout. Most prominently, ME/CFS and autistic burnout are both characterized by severe exhaustion/fatigue and cognitive difficulties (Centers for Disease Control and Prevention, n.d.). Just like ME/CFS, these symptoms can last for years if autistics in burnout remain undiagnosed and continue to expose themselves to perpetuating environmental factors.

However, the etiologies of ME/CFS and autistic burnout are different; autistic burnout has a clear cause related to prolonged stress, demands exceeding capabilities, and a lack of disability-related support.

To differentiate between these conditions, clinicians must gather a thorough history and identify environmental stressors that precipitate and maintain autistic burnout.

Consequences of Autistic Burnout

Negative Impacts

Autistic burnout negatively impacts mental and physical health, the capacity for employment, independent living, and overall quality of life and well-being (Raymaker et al., 2020).

Impacts of autistic burnout on overall functioning include (Mantzalas et al., 2022):

1. Exhaustion and an inability to function
2. Decreased ability to produce and process speech
3. Loss of previously acquired skills (e.g., self-care)
4. Heightened sensitivity to sensory stimuli
5. Reduced executive function (e.g., attention and emotion regulation)

Impacts of autistic burnout on mental health include (Arnold et al., 2023; Richards et al., 2023; Mantzalas et al., 2022):

1. Suicidality
2. Depression
3. Anxiety

Based on the above, we theorize possible secondary impacts of autistic burnout include:

1. Not achieving academic and employment potential
2. Lack of self-fulfillment and self-actualization
3. Relationship difficulties
4. Institutionalization
5. Homelessness

Positive Impacts

Based on our own lived experiences and our work with late-diagnosed autistics, we find that identifying burnout can be a catalyst for undiagnosed autistics to become aware of their identity.

Many undiagnosed adults are unaware that their autistic burnout and general mental health struggles originate from trying to 'live a neurotypical life' as an autistic with different needs and functioning.

When an undiagnosed autistic reaches a crisis point, seeking out support from healthcare professionals may lead to:

1. A formal autism diagnosis
2. Better self-awareness
3. Improved self-care
4. A new perspective on past experiences
5. Increased self-worth
6. Increased self-efficacy
7. Avenues for community support
8. Exploration of self-identity

Prevention and Recovery

Prevention and recovery are the priorities of autistic burnout treatment (Mantzalas, 2022); but for undiagnosed autistic adults, seeking support for autistic burnout may open the door for self-discovery and improved quality of life moving forward.

Conclusion

Autistic burnout is caused by the demands of living in a neurotypical society. Environmental factors, such as social, sensory, daily life, work, and cognitive demands exceed the capacity of many autistic individuals leading to and/or exacerbating autistic burnout—particularly in individuals who have poor mental health, who engage in masking/camouflaging, and who have low self-awareness.

Autistics in autistic burnout experience exhaustion, cognitive and mood changes, withdrawal from social interactions, a heightening of autistic traits, and a reduced ability to mask/camouflage.

Autistics in autistic burnout can recover by removing oneself from contributing causes, resting, identifying areas where changes are needed and support/accommodations are required, engaging in special interests, and gradually reintegrating into society. Recovery is also facilitated by accessing social supports, spending time with fellow autistics, living more authentically (reducing masking/camouflaging), and seeking therapy to improve self-awareness.

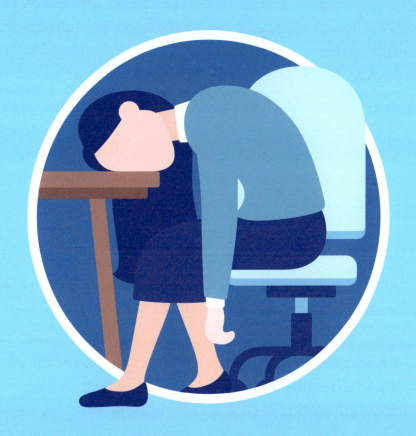

References

1. Autism and Developmental Disabilities Monitoring (ADDM) Network. (2023). Community Reports on Autism 2023. Centers for Disease Control and Prevention. https://www.cdc.gov/ncbddd/autism/pdf/ADDM-Community-Report-SY2020-h.pdf

2. Alaghband-Rad, J., Hajikarim-Hamedani, A., & Motamed, M. (2023). Camouflage and masking behavior in adult autism. Frontiers in psychiatry, 14, 1108110. https://doi.org/10.3389%2Ffpsyt.2023.1108110

3. Alsalhe, T. A., Chalghaf, N., Guelmami, N., Azaiez, F., & Bragazzi, N. L. (2021). Occupational burnout prevalence and its determinants among physical education teachers: A systematic review and meta-analysis. Frontiers in Human Neuroscience, 15, 553230. https://doi.org/10.3389/fnhum.2021.553230

4. Ameri, M., Schur, L., Adya, M., Bentley, F. S., McKay, P. F., & Kruse, D. (2017). The Disability Employment Puzzle: A field experiment on employer hiring behavior. Industrial & Labor Relations Review, 71(2), 329–364. https://doi.org/10.1177/0019793917717474

5. American Psychiatric Association. (2022). Diagnostic and statistical manual of mental disorders (5th ed., text rev.). https://doi.org/10.1176/appi.books.9780890425787

6. Arnold, S., Higgins, J., Weise, J., Desai, A., Pellicano, L., & Trollor, J. (2022). Investigating autistic burnout #AutBurnout: Final Report. (ISBN: 978-1-922365-28–6). Autism CRC. Retrieved July 2, 2024, from https://www.autismcrc.com.au/sites/default/files/reports/3-076RI_Autistic-Burnout_Final-report.pdf

7.   Arnold, S. R., Higgins, J. M., Weise, J., Desai, A., Pellicano, E., & Trollor, J. N. (2023). Towards the measurement of autistic burnout. Autism, 27(7), 1933–1948. https://doi.org/10.1177/13623613221147401

8.   Autism Research Database – Strategic Plan Questions | IACC. (n.d.). iacc.hhs.gov. https://iacc.hhs.gov/funding/data/?fy=2018

9.   Aylward, B. S., Gal-Szabo, D. E., & Taraman, S. (2021). Racial, Ethnic, and Sociodemographic Disparities in Diagnosis of Children with Autism Spectrum Disorder. Journal of Developmental and Behavioral Pediatrics/Journal of Developmental & Behavioral Pediatrics, 42(8), 682–689. https://doi.org/10.1097/dbp.0000000000000996

10. Ayres, M., Parr, J. R., Rodgers, J., Mason, D., Avery, L., & Flynn, D. (2018). A systematic review of quality of life of adults on the autism spectrum. Autism: The International Journal of Research and Practice, 22(7), 774–783. https://doi.org/10.1177/1362361317714988

11. Baron-Cohen, S., Wheelwright, S., Skinner, R., Martin, J., & Clubley, E. (2001). The autism-spectrum quotient (AQ): evidence from Asperger syndrome/high-functioning autism, males and females, scientists and mathematicians. Journal of Autism and Developmental Disorders, 31(1), 5–17. https://doi.org/10.1023/a:1005653411471

12. Beck, A. T., Steer, R. A., & Brown, G. (1996). Beck Depression Inventory–II (BDI-II) [Database record]. APA PsycTests. https://doi.org/10.1037/t00742-000

13. Bemmouna, D., Coutelle, R., Weibel, S. et al. Feasibility, Accept-ability and Preliminary Efficacy of Dialectical Behavior Therapy for Autistic Adults without Intellectual Disability: A Mixed Methods Study. J Autism Dev Disord 52, 4337–4354 (2022). https://doi.org/10.1007/s10803-021-05317-w

14. Bos, J., & Stokes, M. A. (2019). Cognitive empathy moderates the relationship between affective empathy and wellbeing in adolescents with autism spectrum disorder. European Journal of Developmental Psychology, 16(4), 433–446. https://doi.org/10.1080/17405629.2018.1444987

15. Bury, S. M., Spoor, J. R., Hayward, S. M., & Hedley, D. (2022). Supporting the mental health and well-being of autistic and other neurodivergent employees in the work environment. In S. M. Bruyere & A. Colella (Eds.), Neurodiversity in the workplace: Interests, issues, and opportunities (pp. 241–266). Routledge. https://doi.org/10.4324/9781003023616-10

16. Canadian Psychology Association. (2021, July 2). "Psychology Works" Fact Sheet: Workplace Burnout. https://cpa.ca/psychology-works-fact-sheet-workplace-burnout/

17. Centers for Disease Control and Prevention. (n.d.) Myalgic Encephalomyelitis/Chronic Fatigue Syndrome. https://www.cdc.gov/me-cfs/about/index.html

18. Chapman, R., & Botha, M. (2023). Neurodivergence-informed therapy. Developmental Medicine and Child Neurology, 65(3), 310–317. https://doi.org/10.1111/dmcn.15384

19. Chen, M., Su, T., Chen, Y., Hsu, J., Huang, K., Chang, W., Chen, T., & Bai, Y. (2013). Comorbidity of allergic and auto-immune diseases in patients with autism spectrum disorder:

A nationwide population-based study. Research in Autism Spectrum Disorders, 7(2), 205–212. https://doi.org/10.1016/j.rasd.2012.08.008

20. Chen, S., Zhong, X., Jiang, L., Zheng, X., Xiong, Y., Ma, S., Qiu, M., Huo, S., Ge, J., & Chen, Q. (2016). Maternal autoimmune diseases and the risk of autism spectrum disorders in offspring: A systematic review and meta-analysis. Behavioural Brain Research, 296, 61–69. https://doi.org/10.1016/j.bbr.2015.08.035

21. Conner, C. M., Ionadi, A., & Mazefsky, C. A. (2023). Recent Research Points to a Clear Conclusion: Autistic People are Thinking About, and Dying by, Suicide at High Rates. The Pennsylvania Journal on Positive Approaches, 12(3), 69. https://www.ncbi.nlm.nih.gov/pmc/articles/PMC11042491/

22. Cooper, A. A., & Mujtaba, B. G. (2022). Assessment of Workplace Discrimination against Individuals with Autism Spectrum Disorder (ASD). SocioEconomic Challenges (SEC), 6(2). https://doi.org/10.21272/sec.6(2).19-28.2022

23. Cooper, K., Smith, L. G. E., & Russell, A. (2017). Social identity, self-esteem, & mental health in autism. European Journal of Social Psychology, 47(7), 844–854. https://doi.org/10.1002/ejsp.2297

24. D'Cruz, A.-M., Ragozzino, M. E., Mosconi, M. W., Shrestha, S., Cook, E. H., & Sweeney, J. A. (2013). Reduced behavioral flexibility in autism spectrum disorders. Neuropsychology, 27(2), 152–160. https://doi.org/10.1037/a0031721

25. DeFilippis, M. (2018). Depression in Children and Adolescents with Autism Spectrum Disorder. Children, 5(9), 112. https://doi.org/10.3390/children5090112

26. Deloitte. (2022). New report by Deloitte Canada and Auticon Canada finds employment barriers, lack of workplace support for autistic community. https://www2.deloitte.com/ca/en/pages/careers/topics/life-at-deloitte/new-report-by-deloitte-canada-and-auticon-canada-finds-employment-barriers-lack-of-workplace-support-for-autistic-community.html

27. Demetriou, E. A., DeMayo, M. M., & Guastella, A. J. (2019). Executive Function in Autism Spectrum Disorder: History, Theoretical Models, Empirical Findings, and Potential as an Endophenotype. Frontiers in psychiatry, 10, 753. https://doi.org/10.3389/fpsyt.2019.00753

28. Deserno, M. K., Borsboom, D., Begeer, S., Agelink van Rentergem, J. A., Mataw, K., & Geurts, H. M. (2019). Sleep determines quality of life in autistic adults: A longitudinal study. Autism Research: Official Journal of the International Society for Autism Research, 12(5), 794–801. https://doi.org/10.1002/aur.2103

29. De Vries, B. (2021). Autism and the right to a hypersensitivity-friendly workspace. Public Health Ethics, 14(3), 281–287. https://doi.org/10.1093/phe/phab021

30. Dhusia, A. H., Dhaimade, P. A., Jain, A. A., Shemna, S. S., & Dubey, P. N. (2019). Prevalence of Occupational Burnout among Resident Doctors Working in Public Sector Hospitals in Mumbai. Indian Journal of Community Medicine: Official Publication of Indian Association of Preventive & Social Medicine, 44(4), 352–356. https://doi.org/10.4103/ijcm.IJCM_78_19

31. Eaton, C., Roarty, K., Doval, N., Shetty, S., Goodall, K., & Rhodes, S. M. (2023). The prevalence of attention deficit/hyperactivity disorder symptoms in children and adolescents with autism spectrum disorder without intellectual disability: A systematic

review. Journal of Attention Disorders, 27(12), 1360–1376. https://doi.org/10.1177/10870547231177466

32. Fichten, C. S., Schipper, F., Cutler, N. L., & University-College, M. (2005). Does volunteering with children affect attitudes toward adults with disabilities? A Prospective study of Unequal Contact. Rehabilitation Psychology, 50(2), 164–173. https://doi.org/10.1037/0090-5550.50.2.164

33. Fisher, N., Patel, H., van Diest, C., & Spain, D. (2022). Using eye movement desensitisation and reprocessing (EMDR) with autistic individuals: A qualitative interview study with EMDR therapists. Psychology and Psychotherapy: Theory, Research and Practice, 95(4), 1071–1089. https://doi.org/10.1111/papt.12419

34. Fisher, N., van Diest, C., Leoni, M., & Spain, D. (2023). Using EMDR with autistic individuals: A Delphi survey with EMDR therapists. Autism, 27(1), 43–53. https://doi.org/10.1177/13623613221080254

35. Frans, Ö., Rimmö, P., Åberg, L., & Fredrikson, M. (2005). Trauma exposure and post-traumatic stress disorder in the general population. Acta Psychiatrica Scandinavica, 111(4), 291–290. https://doi.org/10.1111/j.1600-0447.2004.00463.x

36. Freudenberger, H. J. (1974). Staff burnout. Journal of social issues, 30(1), 159–165. https://doi.org/10.1111/j.1540-4560.1974.tb00706.x

37. Gaigg, S. B., Flaxman, P. E., McLaven, G., Shah, R., Bowler, D. M., Meyer, B., Roestorf, A., Haenschel, C., Rodgers, J., & South, M. (2020). Self-guided mindfulness and cognitive behavioural practices reduce anxiety in autistic adults: A pilot 8-month waitlist-controlled trial of widely available online tools. Autism, 24(4), 867–883. https://doi.org/10.1177/1362361320909184

38. Hajikarim-Hamedani, A., & Motamed, M. (2023). Camouflage and masking behavior in adult autism. Frontiers in Psychiatry, 14. https://doi.org/10.3389/fpsyt.2023.1108110

39. Harris, L., Gilmore, D., Hanks, C., Coury, D., Moffatt-Bruce, S., Garvin, J. H., & Hand, B. N. (2021). "It was surprisingly equivalent to the appointment I had in person": Advantages and disadvantages of synchronous telehealth for delivering primary care for autistic adults. Autism, 26(6), 1573–1580. https://doi.org/10.1177/13623613211060589

40. Heaton, P. F., Reichenbacher, L., Sauter, D., Allen, R., Scott, S., & Hill, E. L. (2012). Measuring the effects of alexithymia on perception of emotional vocalizations in autistic spectrum disorder and typical development. Psychological Medicine, 42(11), 2453–2459. https://doi.org/10.1017/s0033291712000621

41. Higgins, J. M., Arnold, S. R., Weise, J., Pellicano, E., & Trollor, J. N. (2021). Defining autistic burnout through experts by lived experience: Grounded Delphi method investigating #AutisticBurnout. Autism: the international journal of research and practice, 25(8), 2356–2369. https://doi.org/10.1177/13623613211019858

42. Hollocks, M. J., Lerh, J. W., Magiati, I., Meiser-Stedman, R., & Brugha, T. (2018). Anxiety and depression in adults with autism spectrum disorder: a systematic review and meta-analysis. Psychological Medicine, 49(4), 559–572. https://doi.org/10.1017/s0033291718002283

43. Horowitz, L. M., Snyder, D. J., Boudreaux, E. D., He, J.-P., Harrington, C. J., Cai, J., Claassen, C. A., Salhany, J. E., Dao, T., Chaves, J. F., Jobes, D. A., Merikangas, K. R., Bridge, J. A., & Pao, M. (2020). Validation of the Ask Suicide-Screening Questions

for adult medical inpatients: A brief tool for all ages. Psychosomatics: Journal of Consultation and Liaison Psychiatry, 61(6), 713–722. https://doi.org/10.1016/j.psym.2020.04.008

44. Hosozawa, M., Yamasaki, S., Ando, S., Endo, K., Morimoto, Y., Kanata, S., Fujikawa, S., Cable, N., Iso, H., Hiraiwa-Hasegawa, M., Kasai, K., & Nishida, A. (2023). Lower help-seeking intentions mediate subsequent depressive symptoms among adolescents with high autistic traits: A population-based cohort study. European Child & Adolescent Psychiatry, 32(4), 621–630. https://doi.org/10.1007/s00787-021-01895-3

45. Hossain, M., Khan, N., Sultana, A., Ma, P., McKyer, E. L. J., Ahmed, H. U., & Purohit, N. (2020). Prevalence of comorbid psychiatric disorders among people with autism spectrum disorder: An umbrella review of systematic reviews and meta-analyses. Psychiatry Research, 287, 112922. https://doi.org/10.1016/j.psychres.2020.112922

46. Howlin, P., & Magiati, I. (2017). Autism spectrum disorder. Current Opinion in Psychiatry, 30(2), 69–76. https://doi.org/10.1097/yco.0000000000000308

47. Hudson, C. C., Hall, L., & Harkness, K. L. (2019). Prevalence of Depressive Disorders in Individuals with Autism Spectrum Disorder: a Meta-Analysis. Journal of Abnormal Child Psychology, 47(1), 165–175. https://doi.org/10.1007/s10802-018-0402-1

48. Hull, L., Petrides, K. V., Allison, C., Smith, P., Baron-Cohen, S., Lai, M., & Mandy, W. (2017). "Putting on My Best Normal": Social Camouflaging in Adults with Autism Spectrum Conditions. Journal of Autism and Developmental Disorders, 47(8), 2519–2534. https://doi.org/10.1007/s10803-017-3166-5

49. Hull, L., Mandy, W., Lai, M., Baron-Cohen, S., Allison, C., Smith, P., & Petrides, K. V. (2018). Development and Validation of the Camouflaging Autistic Traits Questionnaire (CAT-Q). Journal of Autism and Developmental Disorders, 49(3), 819–833. https://doi.org/10.1007/s10803-018-3792-6

50. Kent, R., & Simonoff, E. (2017). Prevalence of anxiety in autism spectrum disorders. In Elsevier eBooks (pp. 5–32). https://doi.org/10.1016/b978-0-12-805122-1.00002-8

51. Kinnaird, E., Stewart, C., & Tchanturia, K. (2019). Investigating alexithymia in autism: A systematic review and meta-analysis. European Psychiatry, 55, 80–89. https://doi.org/10.1016/j.eurpsy.2018.09.004

52. Kovács, M., Muity, G., Szapáry, Á., Nemeskéri, Z., Váradi, I., Kapus, K., Tibold, A., Zalayné, N. M., Horvath, L., & Fehér, G. (2023). The prevalence and risk factors of burnout and its association with mental issues and quality of life among Hungarian postal workers: a cross-sectional study. BMC Public Health, 23(1), 75. https://doi.org/10.1186/s12889-023-15002-5

53. Kristensen, T. S., Borritz, M., Villadsen, E., & Christensen, K. B. (2005). The Copenhagen Burnout Inventory: A new tool for the assessment of burnout. Work and Stress, 19(3), 192–207. https://doi.org/10.1080/02678370500297720

54. Linden, A., Best, L., Elise, F., Roberts, D., Branagan, A., Tay, Y. B. E., Crane, L., Cusack, J., Davidson, B., Davidson, I., Hearst, C., Mandy, W., Rai, D., Smith, E., & Gurusamy, K. (2023). Benefits and harms of interventions to improve anxiety, depression, and other mental health outcomes for autistic people: A systematic review and network meta-analysis of randomised controlled trials. Autism, 27(1), 7–30. https://doi.org/10.1177/13623613221117931

55. Lindsay, S., & Cancelliere, S. (2017). A model for developing disability confidence. Disability and Rehabilitation, 40(18), 2122–2130. https://doi.org/10.1080/09638288.2017.1326533

56. Livingston, L. A., Shah, P., & Happé, F. (2019). Compensatory strategies below the behavioural surface in autism: a qualitative study. the Lancet. Psychiatry, 6(9), 766–777. https://doi.org/10.1016/s2215-0366(19)30224-x

57. Lobregt-van Buuren, E., Sizoo, B., Mevissen, L. et al. Eye Movement Desensitization and Reprocessing (EMDR) Therapy as a Feasible and Potential Effective Treatment for Adults with Autism Spectrum Disorder (ASD) and a History of Adverse Events. J Autism Dev Disord 49, 151–164 (2019). https://doi.org/10.1007/s10803-018-3687-6

58. Loomes, R., Hull, L., & Mandy, W. P. L. (2017). What is the Male-to-Female Ratio in Autism Spectrum Disorder? A Systematic Review and Meta-Analysis. Journal of the American Academy of Child and Adolescent Psychiatry, 56(6), 466–474. https://doi.org/10.1016/j.jaac.2017.03.013

59. McCormack, G., Dillon, A. C., Healy, O., Walsh, C., & Lydon, S. (2020). Primary care physicians' knowledge of autism and evidence-based interventions for autism: A systematic review. Review Journal of Autism and Developmental Disorders, 7(3), 226–241. https://doi.org/10.1007/s40489-019-00189-4

60. Addressing employee burnout: Are you solving the right problem? (2022, May 27). McKinsey Health Institute. https://www.mckinsey.com/mhi/our-insights/addressing-employee-burnout-are-you-solving-the-right-problem

61. Maenner MJ, Warren Z, Williams AR, et al. Prevalence and Characteristics of Autism Spectrum Disorder Among Children Aged 8 Years — Autism and Developmental Disabilities Monitoring Network, 11 Sites, United States, 2020. MMWR Surveill Summ 2023;72(No. SS-2):1–14. DOI: http://dx.doi.org/10.15585/mmwr.ss7202a1

62. Mantzalas, J., Richdale, A. L., & Dissanayake, C. (2022). A conceptual model of risk and protective factors for autistic burnout. Autism Research, 15(6), 976–987. https://doi.org/10.1002/aur.2722

63. Mantzalas, J., Richdale, A. L., Li, X., & Dissanayake, C. (2024). Measuring and validating autistic burnout. Autism Research. https://doi.org/10.1002/aur.3129

64. Marco, E. J., Hinkley, L. B., Hill, S. S., & Nagarajan, S. S. (2011). Sensory processing in autism: A review of neurophysiologic findings. Pediatric Research, 69(8), 48–54. https://doi.org/10.1203/PDR.0b013e3182130c54

65. Maslach, C., Jackson, S. E., & Leiter, M. P. (Eds.). (1996). Maslach Burnout Inventory manual (4th ed.). Mind Garden. https://www.mindgarden.com/maslach-burnout-inventory-mbi/685-mbi-manual.html

66. Mattila, A. K., Salminen, J. K., Nummi, T., & Joukamaa, M. (2006). Age is strongly associated with alexithymia in the general population. Journal of Psychosomatic Research, 61(5), 629–635. https://doi.org/10.1016/j.jpsychores.2006.04.013

67. Mazurek, M. O., Pappagianopoulos, J., Brunt, S., Sadikova, E., Nevill, R., Menezes, M., & Harkins, C. (2023). A mixed methods study of autistic adults' mental health therapy experiences. Clinical Psychology & Psychotherapy, 30(4), 767–779. https://doi.org/10.1002/cpp.2835

68. McCrossin, R. (2022). Finding the True Number of Females with Autistic Spectrum Disorder by Estimating the Biases in Initial Recognition and Clinical Diagnosis. Children, 9(2), 272. https://doi.org/10.3390/children9020272

69. Milosavljevic, B., Leno, V. C., Simonoff, E., Baird, G., Pickles, A., Jones, C. R. G., Erskine, C., Charman, T., & Happé, F. (2015). Alexithymia in Adolescents with Autism Spectrum Disorder: Its Relationship to Internalising Difficulties, Sensory Modulation and Social Cognition. Journal of Autism and Developmental Disorders, 46(4), 1354–1367. https://doi.org/10.1007/s10803-015-2670-8

70. Milton, D., Gurbuz, E., & Lopez, B. (2022). The 'double empathy problem': Ten years on. Autism: The International Journal of Research and Practice, 26(8), 1901–1903. https://doi.org/10.1177/13623613221129123

71. Morgan, B., Nageye, F., Masi, G., & Cortese, S. (2020). Sleep in adults with Autism Spectrum Disorder: A systematic review and meta-analysis of subjective and objective studies. Sleep Medicine, 65, 113–120. https://doi.org/10.1016/j.sleep.2019.07.019

72. Newell, V., Phillips, L., Jones, C., Townsend, E., Richards, C., & Cassidy, S. (2023). A systematic review and meta-analysis of suicidality in autistic and possibly autistic people without co-occurring intellectual disability. Molecular autism, 14(1), 12. https://doi.org/10.1186/s13229-023-00544-7

73. Nguyen, W., Ownsworth, T., Nicol, C., & Zimmerman, D. (2020). How I See and Feel About Myself: Domain-Specific Self-Concept and Self-Esteem in Autistic Adults. Frontiers in Psychology, 11, 913. https://doi.org/10.3389/fpsyg.2020.00913

74. Nimmo-Smith, V., Heuvelman, H., Dalman, C., Lundberg, M., Idring, S., Carpenter, P., Magnusson, C., & Rai, D. (2019). Anxiety Disorders in Adults with Autism Spectrum Disorder: A Population-Based Study. Journal of Autism and Developmental Disorders, 50(1), 308–318. https://doi.org/10.1007/s10803-019-04234-3

75. Ontario Human Rights Commission. (n.d.). Policy on ableism and discrimination based on disability: 6. Forms of discrimination. https://www.ohrc.on.ca/en/policy-ableism-and-discrimination-based-disability/6-forms-discrimination

76. Pahnke, J., Jansson-Fröjmark, M., Andersson, G., Bjureberg, J., Jokinen, J., Bohman, B., & Lundgren, T. (2023). Acceptance and commitment therapy for autistic adults: A randomized controlled pilot study in a psychiatric outpatient setting. Autism, 27(5), 1461–1476. https://doi.org/10.1177/13623613221140749

77. Pantazakos, T. (2023). Neurodiversity and psychotherapy—Connections and ways forward. Counselling and Psychotherapy Research. https://doi.org/10.1002/capr.12675

78. Phou, A. K. (2019). The Effects of Diaphragmatic Breathing on Anxiety in Children with High Functioning Autism Spectrum Disorder: A Pilot Study. California State University, Long Beach. ProQuest. https://www.proquest.com/openview/f59051e5e853aaaeb4ab8052af37ce4c/1

79. Posserud, M., Solberg, B. S., Engeland, A., Haavik, J., & Klungsøyr, K. (2021). Male to female ratios in autism spectrum disorders by age, intellectual disability and attention-deficit/hyperactivity disorder. Acta Psychiatrica Scandinavica, 144(6), 635–646. https://doi.org/10.1111/acps.13368

80. Quadt, L., Williams, G., Mulcahy, J., Larsson, D. E. O., Silva, M., Arnold, A. J., Critchley, H., & Garfinkel, S. N. (2023). "I'm trying to reach out, I'm trying to find my people": A Mixed-Methods investigation of the link between sensory differences, loneliness, and mental health in autistic and nonautistic adults. Autism in Adulthood. https://doi.org/10.1089/aut.2022.0062

81. Rai, D., Culpin, I., Heuvelman, H., Magnusson, C. M. K., Carpenter, P., Jones, H. J., Emond, A. M., Zammit, S., Golding, J., & Pearson, R. M. (2018). Association of Autistic Traits With Depression From Childhood to Age 18 Years. JAMA psychiatry, 75(8), 835–843. https://doi.org/10.1001/jamapsychiatry.2018.1323

82. Raymaker, D. M., Teo, A. R., Steckler, N. A., Lentz, B., Scharer, M., Delos Santos, A., Kapp, S. K., Hunter, M., Joyce, A., & Nicolaidis, C. (2020). "Having all of your internal resources exhausted beyond measure and being left with no clean-up crew": Defining Autistic Burnout. Autism in Adulthood: challenges and management, 2(2), 132–143. https://doi.org/10.1089/aut.2019.0079

83. Reuben, K., Stanzione, C. M., & Singleton, J. L. (2021). Interpersonal trauma and posttraumatic stress in autistic adults. Autism in Adulthood, 3(3), 247–256. https://doi.org/10.1089/aut.2020.0073

84. Richards, J. K., McKenney, E. E., Day, T., & Lerner, M. D. (2023). The reliability and validity of a novel autistic burnout measure among neurodiverse college students. ResearchGate. https://www.researchgate.net/publication/370632959_The_Reliability_and_Validity_of_a_Novel_Autistic_Burnout_Measure_Among_Neurodiverse_College_Students

85. Ritvo, R. A., Ritvo, E. R., Guthrie, D., Ritvo, M. J., Hufnagel, D. H., McMahon, W., Tonge, B., Mataix-Cols, D., Jassi, A., Attwood, T., & Eloff, J. (2010). Ritvo Autism Asperger Diagnostic Scale–Revised (RAADS–R) [Database record]. APA PsycTests. https://doi.org/10.1037/t06014-000

86. Roberts, A. L., Koenen, K. C., Lyall, K., Robinson, E. B., & Weisskopf, M. G. (2015). Association of autistic traits in adulthood with childhood abuse, interpersonal victimization, and post-traumatic stress. Child Abuse & Neglect, 45, 135–142. https://pubmed.ncbi.nlm.nih.gov/25957197/

87. Rommelse, N. N. J., Franke, B., Geurts, H. M., Hartman, C. A., & Buitelaar, J. K. (2010). Shared heritability of attention-deficit/hyperactivity disorder and autism spectrum disorder. European Child & Adolescent Psychiatry, 19(3), 281–295. https://doi.org/10.1007/s00787-010-0092-x

88. Rumball, F., Happé, F., & Grey, N. (2020). Experience of trauma and PTSD symptoms in autistic adults: Risk of PTSD development following DSM-5 and Non-DSM-5 traumatic life events. Autism Research, 13(12), 2122–2132. https://doi.org/10.1002/aur.2306

89. Salminen, J. K., Saarijärvi, S., Äärelä, E., Toikka, T., & Kauhanen, J. (1999). Prevalence of alexithymia and its association with sociodemographic variables in the general population of finland. Journal of Psychosomatic Research, 46(1), 75–82. https://doi.org/10.1016/s0022-3999(98)00053-1

90. Shenouda, J., Barrett, E., Davidow, A. L., Sidwell, K., Lescott, C., Halperin, W., Silenzio, V. M. B., & Zahorodny, W. (2023). Prevalence & disparities in the detection of autism without intellectual disability. Pediatrics, 151(2). https://doi.org/10.1542/peds.2022-056594

91. Stewart, T. M., Martin, K., Fazi, M., Oldridge, J., Piper, A., & Rhodes, S. (2021). A systematic review of the rates of depression in autistic children and adolescents without intellectual disability. Psychology and Psychotherapy, 95(1), 313–344. https://doi.org/10.1111/papt.12366

92. Tomczak, M. T., & Kulikowski, K. (2023). Toward an understanding of occupational burnout among employees with autism – the Job Demands-Resources theory perspective. Current Psychology, 43(2), 1582–1594. https://doi.org/10.1007/s12144-023-04428-0

93. Vasa, R. A., Keefer, A., McDonald, R. G., Hunsche, M. C., & Kerns, C. M. (2020). A Scoping Review of Anxiety in Young Children with Autism Spectrum Disorder. Autism Research, 13(12), 2038–2057. https://doi.org/10.1002/aur.2395

94. Warrier, V., Greenberg, D. M., Weir, E., Buckingham, C., Smith, P., Lai, M., & Allison, C. (2020). Elevated rates of autism, other neurodevelopmental and psychiatric diagnoses, and autistic traits in transgender and gender-diverse individuals. Nature Communications, 11(1), 1–12. https://doi.org/10.1038/s41467-020-17794-1

95. Whitney, D. G., & Shapiro, D. N. (2019). National prevalence of pain among children and adolescents with autism spectrum disorders. JAMA pediatrics, 173(12), 1203–1205. https://doi.org/10.1001/jamapediatrics.2019.3826

96. Winn, B. (2015). WARC's Guidelines for Interviewing Autistic Individuals. Wales Autism Research Centre, The University of Cardiff. https://www.autistica.org.uk/downloads/files/Guidelines-for-interviewing-by-Beverley-Winn-et-al.pdf

97. World Health Organization (2019). International Statistical Classification of Diseases and Related Health Problems (11th ed.). https://icd.who.int/en

98. World Health Organization. (2023, March 31). Depressive disorder (depression). https://www.who.int/news-room/fact-sheets/detail/depression

99. Zeidan, J., Fombonne, E., Scorah, J., Ibrahim, A., Durkin, M. S., Saxena, S., Yusuf, A., Shih, A., & Elsabbagh, M. (2022). Global prevalence of autism: A systematic review update. Autism Research, 15(5), 778–790. https://doi.org/10.1002/aur.2696

Non-Clinical Version

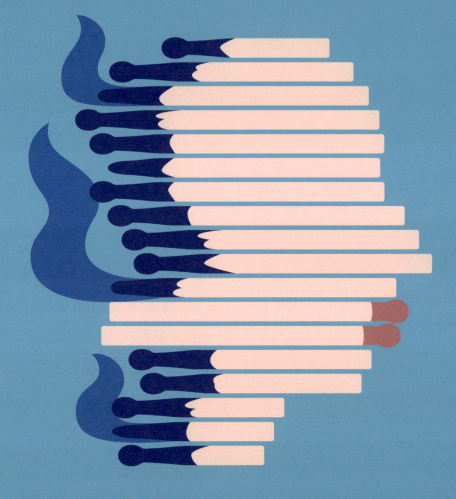

The next section of this book features a more accessible rewriting of the clinical version, with more comprehensive explanations and links to external sources for more information.

What is Autistic Burnout?

Autistic burnout (ABO) is a widely discussed and experienced condition among autistics. In the simplest terms, autistic burnout is a state of complete exhaustion caused by existing in a non-autistic world.[1]

Autistics—in research—describe the experience of autistic burnout as chronic exhaustion, loss of skills, and reduced tolerance to stimuli. It is caused by long-term stress and tasks that overwhelm an autistic's capacity. It affects all areas of an autistic's life and can lead to a loss of relationships, jobs, and mental and physical wellbeing.

One of the most frustrating aspects of autistic burnout is the lack of clinician awareness of autism coupled with managing the autistic burnout itself. Many autistics report experiencing **impostor syndrome** regarding their autism and autistic burnout. They feel that they are just being lazy or just not trying hard enough.

We need the external world to validate our internal experiences in order to feel confidence and internal validation.

An example from Natalie:

> For a long time, I struggled with feeling unlikeable. The problem was surrounding myself with individuals who criticized me for who I was. After being diagnosed as autistic, I began spending time with those who value me for who I am, and that external validation allowed me to realize that I am likable.

It is essential to have someone acknowledge our experiences. Recognition can be as simple as "I see that this is real and that you are going through it." It's crucial to become well-acquainted with the signs and symptoms of autistic burnout. We must understand what it looks like, its causes, and how to provide appropriate support.

The presentation of the majority of autistics is largely misunderstood. Many people are unaware that at least **66%** of autistics are without intellectual disability or language disability.[2] The medical field requires remembering large amounts of information and systemizing that information. These are common strengths of autistics, and as such, many autistics are our healthcare providers.

Yet, studies have shown that autistic doctors are highly suicidal, with **77%** experiencing suicidal ideation and almost half (**49%**) self-harming.[3] Many do not disclose being autistic, as their colleagues carry the false belief that autistic people cannot be doctors. This is due to the research focusing on the deficits and difficulties of having autism rather than the differences and gifts that come with being autistic.

If our healthcare providers are unaware of how autism presents and unaware that many of their colleagues are autistic, what hope do autistic people in general have of being identified as autistic and receiving the help they need? The time has come for us to challenge this pathologizing perspective and begin to examine autism in its entirety.

In autistic burnout research, much of the initial research stems from online discussions about the shared experience of autistic burnout. At present, there is no official medical diagnosis for autistic burnout. Autistics, with their friends and families, are left to search for answers about this debilitating condition.

Neither autistic burnout nor occupational burnout are listed in the **DSM-5**. However, the **World Health Organization** has included occupational burnout in the **ICD-11**, and the **DSM-5-TR** is considering including it in the next edition. With more research and information on autistic burnout, we hope it will follow a similar trajectory and eventually find its way in diagnostic manuals.

Even though autistic burnout is not listed within the current version of the diagnostic manuals, it does not mean that it is not a valid and real condition. Conditions generally require a significant amount of time to enter the disease classification manuals. For example, occupational burnout was first identified in 1973, but has yet to be included in the DSM.

Similarly, conditions such as **pathological demand avoidance** (PDA), **Internet addiction disorder** (IAD), **sex addiction, complex post-traumatic stress disorder** (C-PTSD), **sensory processing disorder** (SPD), and **misophonia**—among others—are also not listed.

Some conditions are in omission because the topic is early in the research or because the panel has decided that another diagnosis covers the condition adequately. In addition, there may be political factors and ethical considerations for not including certain constructs at a given time.

Our solution is to write a series of books educating patients and healthcare providers on autism-related topics. Many general practitioners may be unaware of autistic burnout despite the fact that it is a common issue for autistics, and it is increasingly covered in the research literature.

If you have a good relationship with your doctor and they are unfamiliar with autistic burnout, you can provide them with a copy of this book; it will give them more opportunities to offer you the treatment and guidance you need to recover from autistic burnout. When people become aware of autistic burnout, a discussion can begin with doctors, friends, and family.

Prevalence Rates

Prevalence of Autistic Burnout

Published data indicates the occurrence of autistic burnout is **69%**, with a high rate of recurrence.[4] Estimates are that **46%** of autistics have had autistic burnout four or more times in their life.

→ A later diagnosis increases the risk of autistic burnout[5]

→ The gender and racial differences of autistic burnout are not currently known

Prevalence of Autism

National Estimates

The prevalence of autism is generally stated to be around **2.5%**; but this will vary per country. As of 2020, the **CDC** has identified the prevalence to be **2.8%** in the US;[6] and in Canada, the prevalence is estimated to be **2%**.[7]

Global Estimates

The estimated global prevalence rate is **0.01–4.36%**.[8] This wide range is due to the great variety in reported autism prevalence for each country; there are differences in how many people seek assessments, differences in diagnostic criteria or their clinical application, differences in data collection and research methods, and possibly racial differences as well.

Gender Ratio

While it is commonly believed that autism occurs more in males than females, research suggests that the timing of diagnoses is relevant, as females tend to get diagnosed later in life.[9]

Accordingly, the difference in prevalence between males and females shrinks in adulthood. The male-to-female ratio for children aged 4–10 is **4.5:1**; but once adulthood is reached, the male-to-female ratio decreases to **2.6:1**.[9]

That is not to say that the **2.6:1** ratio is accurate, as it may still reflect a gender bias in autism diagnoses; cultural perceptions of autism and differences in presentation may lead to males being assessed and diagnosed more readily than females.

Diagnostic Gender Bias

The male-to-female ratio of autism has shifted from **4:1** to **3:1** over the years, which shows a gender bias in autism diagnoses.[10]

Some estimate that the true male-to-female ratio may be closer to **2:1**; but research from 2022 using a mathematical model based on published data of autism diagnoses indicates that the true ratio may even be **3:4**; and that **80%** of females remain undiagnosed at age 18.[11]

BIPOC Individuals

Although previously, BIPOC people were diagnosed later in life than Caucasians, due to advocacy, research is now showing that Black, Hispanic, and Asian children are actually diagnosed earlier than white children on average. Roughly **3%** of Black, Hispanic, and Asian or Pacific Islander children are diagnosed as autistic, compared to about **2%** of white children.[12]

There is a lot to be said about autism diagnoses for BIPOC individuals and how it relates to stigma and discrimination. We hope to explore this topic further in a future book.

Causes

Autistic burnout is caused by the challenges that autistic people face living in a non-autistic world. In order to be understood and prevent ostracization, autistic people are required to behave in a non-autistic manner.[13, 14] Research shows that non-autistics identify that something is different and therefore aversive about an autistic within two minutes of meeting them.[15, 16] To prevent these negative consequences, autistics often feel forced to camouflage their autistic traits. In other words, autistics are forced to hide their proclivities and engage in activities that are objectionable to them in order to feel included.

Research suggests that non-autistics use facial expressions for different purposes than autistics. For example, due to sensitivity to face processing, autistics do not use eye contact to emphasize points in their speech, while non-autistics do.[17] There are also differences in body language and speech patterns, making the two neurotypes foreign to each other.[18] When an autistic person interacts with a non-autistic (allistic/neurotypical) person, they must use speech and non-verbal communication patterns that mimic non-autistics to be understood.

The majority of the world does not communicate in the same way as autistic people; and as such, it has been autistics who have had to learn to adapt and mimic neurotypical speech and behaviour. The mimicking does not mean that the autistic person inherently understands it, however. This can lead to further misunderstanding and miscommunication, and more expenditure of energy—without guaranteed success in communication.

So there is a disproportional expenditure of energy and cognitive effort for autistic people to understand others and make themselves understood. This can eventually lead to autistic burnout.

Research in 2019 showed that those with higher autistic traits make better armchair social psychologists.[19] We are good at predicting the meaning of behaviours we have seen previously. However, we experience challenges once the context changes, as we may not realize that the same behaviour has a different meaning.

For example, we discussed how an autistic may have learned that "Hi, how are you?" is not a question but a greeting; however, within the context of therapy, it becomes a genuine question. It is challenging for an autistic to understand this difference.

Around **94–98%** of the world consists of non-autistic individuals,[7, 8] and therefore, the world largely does not speak the same 'language' as us. We are put in a position of having to translate body language, context, and implied meanings from a non-autistic language into an autistic language. Then, we must translate it back to answer. This takes time and energy.

In addition, there is an environmental challenge. An autistic brain is designed to pick up far more sensory data. An environment that feels comfortable to a non-autistic can be extremely uncomfortable to an autistic—it can be too loud, too bright, or overwhelming with smells. The environmental problem along with the "language barrier" is exhausting and thus contributes to large amounts of energy consumption in autistics, just to function in an environment that is comfortable for a non-autistic.

An easy example is to imagine a fish out of water. It would be silly to think that there is something wrong with a fish for not being able to breathe out of water—they are simply in an unfitting environment.

Autistics need context and are altogether literal. An example is a patient who shared that their boss said, "Now photocopying needs to be done." This autistic person did not do the photocopying because their boss did not tell them to do it—just that it had to be done. A fair assumption from an autistic perspective is that the task had yet to be delegated. After being reprimanded, they learned that their boss meant for them to be the one to do the photocopying.

These factors and others cause chronic life stress for autistics. In addition to the environment and expectations from others, autistics can put tremendous pressure on themselves. It is common for them to enthusiastically overestimate what is possible for them to do versus what they are capable of doing. This mismatch between their expectations and their abilities can lead to autistic burnout.

1. Social Demands

To autistics, social demands are obligations and expectations. These demands often take them away from activities that provide them with energy, such as their special interests. Engaging socially can be draining for autistics, regardless of whether they enjoy the activity or not. Even enjoyable experiences can be tiring for them. Initiating, engaging, and terminating social experiences are often confusing irrespective of whether they must mask their true selves.

Social demands are overwhelming because we typically have little extra time to devote to social interactions and demands. Autistic individuals derive energy from being alone, sticking to their routines, and pursuing their passionate interests. They are known for excellence in their work. They pay exceptional attention to detail and are incredible problem-solvers; however, they must be able to devote their time to their pursuits.

About a young autistic woman (age 24):

An adult autistic who wanted to learn Spanish became so proficient that she was mistaken for a native speaker within just seven months, all while working a demanding full-time job. In school, she was excellent at math but struggled with language, yet she was so dedicated to this pursuit that she was able to accomplish it.

During this time, she withdrew from all social relationships and spent very little time engaging with others. She described that all social requirements pulled her away from her learning, which she experienced as exceedingly frustrating during this time.

Most adults cannot become proficient in a second language beyond a certain age; research has indicated that to achieve grammatical fluency comparable to that of a native speaker, one should aim to do so by age 18, with the ideal starting age being 10. Our excellence in our work comes from the time we invest in our interests. Because of this, those we are closest to are often people who share our passions.

To produce excellence in our pursuits—be it work or a video game— the autistic must exert an inordinate amount of time. The autistic brain is driven to want to do our preferred activities. For example:

Natalie:

The idea behind this book started as a pamphlet, which then grew to a booklet, and has now become a 228-page book. I had to be told by someone that I must enforce a limit to the otherwise endless growth of the project.

The concept of 'getting together to chit-chat' can be overwhelming; there is no time or space for it. Once we have something initiated, it is extremely difficult to stop. The research literature refers to this as 'inertial motion', which is part of so-called autistic inertia.[19] Irrespective of who is being engaged with, the interaction will require significant energy. It does not mean that we don't like social engagement.

For instance, someone might enjoy driving a car, but they'll still run out of gas or get tired eventually. Moreover, there are certain activities that are even more demanding, such as engaging with a non-autistic. This requires a particularly high energetic cost due to camouflaging.

Camouflaging is a powerful evolutionary tactic used by many animals to disguise their appearance in order to avoid detection or to imitate other animals so as to deter predators. Similarly, social camouflaging refers to the strategies autistics use to blend into their social surroundings. We change ourselves to present as different from who we are. We use this tactic to be perceived in a way that is deemed 'appropriate' by the group(s) (the non-autistics) we want to be included in.

For non-autistics, camouflaging might mean acting, talking, and/or dressing in a certain way in order to fit in with their preferred social group. This need also applies to autistic individuals; however, our need to camouflage goes deeper—it involves hiding our autistic traits in order to minimize the visibility of our autism in social situations.

As mentioned earlier, non-autistic individuals can often sense that something is different (and therefore aversive) about us within just two minutes of interacting. For an autistic person, camouflaging becomes a matter of social survival when living in a non-autistic world.

The reasons for camouflaging can be grouped into three categories:

1. Conventional
2. Relational
3. Other

Conventional

Conventional reasons for camouflaging include communicating our ideas or work, performing well in our job or university, collaborating effectively with peers, getting others to take us or our ideas seriously, reducing awkwardness in social situations, demonstrating responsibility, and obtaining promotions.

Relational

Relationally, we camouflage our traits to make it easier to form friendships, attract potential romantic partners, seem more likable, bond with others, fit in, demonstrate success and trustworthiness, and express intelligence.

Other

Beyond that, we also mask to fit into a neurotypical world, avoid retaliation and bullying, and manage the impression others have of us.

Many of us have an internalized stigma regarding our autistic traits to the extent that camouflaging becomes such a deeply-ingrained habit that we may not even realize we are doing it.

Mutual Mismatch in Communication

Communication between autistics and non-autistics can be challenging at times. The 'double empathy' concept (read more about this on the next page) highlights the challenge of autistics and non-autistics in understanding each other.[21] This mutual misunderstanding can make autistics feel othered and left out.

Environments dominated by cross-neurotype communication can lead to burnout, as they demand a lot more energy, effort, and focus to sustain effective communication, respond appropriately to social situations, and meet social and communication-based expectations.

Autistic individuals are often assumed to have deficits in social and communication skills because they communicate differently from the non-autistic majority. This perspective is highly neuro-normative, as it presumes that the dominant form of communication is superior simply because it's the most common. The so-called 'dialectical misattunement hypothesis' more comprehensively describes this mutual mismatch or misattunement in communication between autistic and non-autistic individuals.[22]

Autistics' direct and less subtle communication style may sometimes appear rude or abrasive to non-autistics. However, it's important to remember that this directness is generally a communication difference—not a sign of disrespect. There is usually no intended subtext, and any intended meaning will be explicitly stated. Understanding this can foster empathy and better communication.

Natalie:

When I ask my (autistic) partner to unload the dishwasher, I say, "Unload the dishwasher." My partner finds this a good way of communicating, as they find it direct and clear; whereas my eldest son—who is non-autistic—says that he finds it very rude.

The Double Empathy Problem

'Double empathy' is a term coined by autistic researcher Damian Milton, used to explain the challenges in understanding between autistics and non-autistics, who have different forms of communication and cognitive styles.[21]

Non-autistics use facial expressions and eye contact to emphasize their words and engage in social interaction. On the other hand, autistics tend to speak and/or use words to convey information, usually to people who share an interest or with whom they need to share information. Both autistics and non-autistics are prosocial (meaning social behaviour that benefits other people or society as a whole—such as helping, sharing, co-operating, volunteering, etc.), but their methods differ.

For instance, while non-autistics perceive flirting as a nuanced interaction, in the autistic world, unless you are direct, all the batting of eyes and subtle flirtation will be for nothing, as autistic people will likely not pick up on this non-verbal communication.

The Triple Empathy Problem

The 'triple empathy problem' explains that healthcare providers who are not trained in communicating with autistics are unaware of what autistics are trying to get across. Healthcare providers typically expect autistics to communicate in non-autistic ways, and with medical terminology. Therefore, there are two levels of disconnect.[24]

Having to use neurotypical communication when speaking to non-autistics can be exhausting for autistics, which can lead to burnout.

Natalie:

> An autistic friend of mine had difficulty expressing to their therapist that they needed help with their anxiety. Each time they went to the appointment, the therapist would ask them how they were. It was confusing to my friend how to bring up their anxiety, which was something they had tried to communicate for months.
>
> I explained that when a therapist says, "Hi, how are you?" they are inquiring about the reason for the visit, not just greeting you.
>
> The struggle to understand expected behaviours in different situations can be very confusing for autistics, who are heavily reliant on context to understand social cues.

2. Sensory Demands

Many autistic individuals experience hypersensitivity to sensory input.[24] Exposure to fluorescent lights, strong smells, loud sounds or other sensory experiences can be distressing or painful for us, impacting our overall well-being and contributing to autistic burnout.[25]

Our senses are what we use to experience the world. We use our senses to gather information about the surroundings through the detection of stimuli. So what is it like to be hypersensitive to common everyday experiences? It is difficult for a person to imagine something they don't experience, and it is a different experience entirely to be bombarded by the stimuli at all times.

For instance, while one could imagine that a dog can hear sounds outside of their normal human range, it doesn't register as we are walking around. Non-autistics walking through a store are not hearing the buzz of electricity, feeling sick from the fluorescent lighting, feeling overwhelmed from the sounds, and so on. As the majority of people are non-autistic, the world is not designed to be sensory-friendly to autistic individuals.

Natalie's internal experience in a part of her day:

My morning sleep is impacted by my dog and the sound of my partner breathing or being in bed. The heat, smells, and sounds begin aggravating me. After getting out of bed, the sensation of the floor under my feet can negatively impact me. I must decide whether to shower or not—if I shower, I will become wet, which is an unpleasant situation.

Once I have showered, it is more difficult to get dressed, as the clothes cling to my wet skin, which bothers me. When getting dressed, I can only wear one type of underwear, which I have worn since age 16. I cannot wear socks, including in the winter. I choose between four dresses that are all from the same company and all made from a particular bamboo fabric, as I cannot tolerate any other materials.

Should I decide to shower, there must be two towels in the bathroom; one to wrap around myself, and one to wrap around my shoulders. I brush my teeth before showering and can only tolerate one type of toothpaste. I must wear sandals. I insist on having an indoor and an outdoor pair of shoes as I cannot be barefoot.

Next, I make breakfast. I drink the same smoothie daily in the summer; it must be the perfect temperature. It must be colder than room temperature, but if it is too cold, it is painful to consume. This is the first 30 minutes of my day—every day—and it continues in the same form. Other people clearly do not experience what I experience, as demonstrated by my recent stay at a 4-star hotel. I encountered several sensory issues during my stay:

On the first day, I had to request a room change due to two reasons. Firstly, someone was smoking in another room, which was causing me headaches. Secondly, there was noise from a band playing 18 floors below me, the sound of which was causing me ear pain.

At that point, I had already managed the fact that the hotel staff had failed to clean up a pair of panties from below my pillow, as well as a used Q-tip and hairpin in my bed. I did not request to move rooms based on the cleanliness exclusively, due to the stress I knew it would cause me. However, when I finally did request to change rooms, I cited the lack of cleanliness as the reason because I felt like I would otherwise be considered a bother, given that no one else seemed to be affected by the noise or smoke.

It is important to remember that:

1. We automatically think everyone experiences the world in the same way as us; this is a natural inclination.

2. Autistics then learn that this is not correct. We learn that we are different. Unfortunately, this difference can make non-autistics believe we are too sensitive, too much, etc.

3. The autistic brain does not gate and remove sensory information. It doesn't habituate sensory information. We receive it all the time at all hours of the day. Most people can relate to the overwhelming odour of walking through the perfume section of a store. However, what most don't realize is that it is how everything is for us—all the time.

3. Cognitive Demands

Autistic individuals find it challenging to adapt to changes in cognitive demands. For instance, we have challenges with certain executive skills, including behavioural flexibility, planning, and working memory.

Executive skills

Executive skills are cognitive processes—a set of mental skills—that allow us to achieve our goals; they help us solve problems, make decisions, and control our actions and behaviours.

Executive functions are primarily regulated in our brain's prefrontal cortex. However, autistic people have altered neural processes that impact how our brain manages these executive functions.

Some of the executive challenges we face necessitates greater cognitive effort, and thus a greater expenditure of energy. This could ultimately contribute to autistic burnout.

Low flexibility

Research also shows that autistics tend to struggle with behavioural flexibility.[26] This partially explains why so many of us adhere to routines and prefer sameness. For example, our challenges with behavioural flexibility means that a last-minute change to our plans can cause extreme distress. Low flexibility can also look like eating the same foods daily for breakfast or seeking comfort by watching our favourite movies repeatedly.

While low flexibility results in difficulty coping with some situations, it is important to note that it is not the case for all situations. There isn't anything "wrong" with wanting to watch an old movie instead of a new one. Context matters!

Rumination

Research also shows that autistics have more negative and unwanted thoughts than non-autistics—especially *brooding* (continuously comparing one's current condition to one's desired condition).[27] Autistics who reported higher levels of obsessive thinking—such as more negative and unwanted thoughts—also reported increased levels of repetitive behaviour.

We conclude that some repetitive behaviours may be linked to anxiety, although further research is required to better understand repetitive behaviours in autism.

Change

Significant or continuous change—causing disruptions in our routines and undermining the level of comfort we find in knowing what to expect—can contribute to autistic burnout. Autistic individuals struggle with change and often manage their stress through sameness, routine, rituals, and predictable patterns.

The distress or burnout caused by changes is not necessarily tied to negative outcomes or events, but rather to the change itself—which can be overwhelming for autistic individuals.

For example:

1. **'Small' changes in routine:** taking a different route; eating a different meal; unexpected greetings; wearing a different pair of shoes; cancelling or rescheduling plans; misplacing an item.

2. **'Large' changes in routine:** starting or leaving a job; beginning a school semester; moving to a new home; getting a pet; losing a valuable item; transitioning from high school to university; welcoming a newborn into the family.

3. **Changes in relationships:** dating someone new; making a new friend; experiencing a break-up; getting a new boss; grieving the loss of a person.

Note

The impact of changes is subjective.
While this list provides common examples,
it is not exhaustive and may not reflect the
experiences of all autistic individuals.

---

4. Daily Life Demands

Managing daily tasks can take a significant toll, and can eventually lead to burnout.

Natalie:

> Many autistics have shared with me that they have difficulty managing to brush their teeth or take a shower. Both activities have a sensory aspect as well as an energy demand.

> Neurotypicals may consider some of these daily tasks annoying, boring, or tiring. For autistics, these tasks can be overwhelming and exhausting.

The combination of executive challenges, social and sensory differences, and tasks that are often considered 'errands' or weekly 'to-dos' by neurotypicals can demand a lot of effort and energy for autistic individuals to manage.

Some examples of daily life demands include:

- Going to the grocery store or other shopping experiences
- Paying bills or doing taxes
- Filling in forms or other administrative work
- Navigating public transit, driving, or reading maps
- Ordering food at a restaurant or leaving a restaurant at the end of a meal
- Going to medical appointments or getting haircuts
- Preparing meals that require many simultaneous steps, a variety of ingredients or cooking methods

5. Insufficient Support

Autistic individuals often experience burnout due to a lack of support, inclusion, accessibility, and accommodations.[28]

Autism is considered a developmental disability, which means autistic people benefit from ongoing support. However, for many, it is an invisible disability; meaning that unlike physical disabilities, autism does not necessarily become apparent to other people—at least not on sight.

Research has shown us that many autistics are doctors—a fact that might be surprising to someone lacking the understanding of how autism presents. See the quote below from the cross-sectional study on the experiences of autistic doctors:[29]

> "Some receive a diagnosis following difficulties in stressful clinical environments, or highly demanding career paths—and that support from employers, including occupational health and professional supervisors is inconsistent, with some colleagues refusing to believe a qualified doctor could be autistic."

Living in a neurotypical-dominant world makes it difficult to access the necessary support. Healthcare professionals—not fully understanding how autism presents—might struggle to provide appropriate accommodations.

This general lack of awareness and accommodations for autism creates constant demands that can overwhelm autistic individuals.[5]

Things that can lead to inadequate support:

- Disbelief from others when you ask for help.

- Feeling invalidated and not being seen or heard.

- Lack of social connections and a sense of belonging, leading to loneliness, which is more distressing for autistic individuals.[30]

- Feeling exhausted and lacking energy.

- Dealing with additional cognitive and emotional burdens.

- Low self-worth and feeling inferior.

- Self-criticism and a lack of self-compassion, feeling incapable but pressuring yourself to meet certain expectations.

- Comparing your experiences to those of non-autistic individuals and holding yourself to the same standards.

- Facing negative judgments and social rejection.

- Lack of awareness about autism at schools, home, or work.[31]

6. Workplace Discrimination

Many autistic individuals face discrimination in the workplace.[32] This discrimination can be direct, such as receiving ableist comments (prejudice based on physical or mental disabilities) or being denied necessary accommodations.

But workplace discrimination can also be indirect, such as being passed over for promotions or opportunities without valid work-related reasons, solely because of being autistic.[33]

Discrimination can also look like employers deliberately changing working conditions just to make it harder for autistics to cope, all in an attempt to make autistic employees leave.

Coworkers can be distant to autistic people, exclude them, or otherwise show discriminating attitudes.[34, 35]

Workplace discrimination can even happen in the hiring process. Research indicates that job applicants who disclose disabilities like autism receive **26%** fewer expressions of interest from potential employers.[36]

For more information on discrimination in the workplace, have a look at the 'Potential consequences for disclosing [autism]' section of our article on workplace accommodations for autistics and those with AuDHD.

Search for 'workplace' on our website (**Embrace-Autism.com**), and the article below should come up.

Workplace accommodations for autism & AuDHD

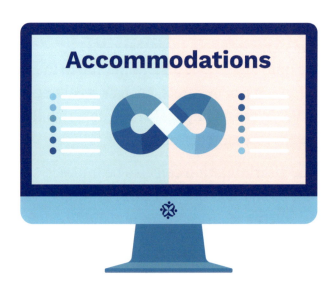

Risk Factors for Autistic Burnout

Although burnout is generally caused by things in the person's environment, some specific traits or characteristics can make autistics more susceptible to burnout. Such traits can not only lead to more stress, but it can also lead to a greater likelihood of getting into stressful environments and relationships.

The following traits, in particular, can lead to autistic burnout:

1. **A lack of self-awareness** (e.g., not being aware of your needs or limitations)

2. **Camouflaging/masking** (which can be very draining over time)

3. **Poor mental health** (which can make it more challenging to cope with things)

4. **Challenges with executive functions** (e.g., organization, planning, time management, attention, and flexibility)

5. **A history of trauma** (which can cause certain triggers and make it more difficult to cope or stay in control of your emotions)

6. **Sensory sensitivities** (can cause overwhelm, which is draining and can result in meltdowns and shutdowns)

1. Low Self-Awareness

When someone has low self-awareness, they struggle to understand their own thoughts and feelings or how others may perceive them. Low self-awareness is often caused by **alexithymia**. Between **50–85%** of autistic people have alexithymia.[37, 38, 39, 40]

People with alexithymia often struggle to recognize, identify, classify, or describe their feelings and sensations.

Many with alexithymia cannot tell the difference between pain and fatigue or hunger and anxiety. Typically, they can only express how they feel in general or vague terms such as sad, "fine", good, and bad.

Low self-awareness leads autistics to burnout by:

- Making it more difficult to recognize stress, distress, pain, or discomfort.

- Making it more challenging to identify and recognize your needs.

- Increasing how well you tolerate pain and distress, because it is outside of your awareness. While this has its benefits in the moment, it can make it difficult to recognize and prevent pain and distress, meaning you will continue to endure more of it until you cannot take any more.

- Not being able to properly report the level of pain or distress you are in, because of low awareness or difficulties with describing the severity of your pain or distress.

- Seeing negative experiences as neutral or even positive, which thus prevents you from avoiding (certain) negative experiences.

2. Camouflaging/Masking

Camouflaging describes strategies some autistics use to better deal with social situations. They use it to fit in, create connections, prevent being rejected by others, or to be accepted by others.[13, 14] Camouflaging takes a lot of energy, which is why it can often lead to burnout, depression, and anxiety in autistics.[15]

Research shows that autistics use three forms of camouflaging:[14]

1. **Compensation:** Used to overcome difficulties in social situations. This involves copying body language and facial expressions, learning social cues from movies and books, and using pre-planned social scripts to make social communication smoother.

2. **Masking:** Involves concealing autistic traits to appear non-autistic. Examples include forcing eye contact and presenting calm facial expressions and body posture to appear confident or relaxed.

3. **Assimilation:** Strategies used to try to fit in with others in social situations. This may include putting on an act, avoiding or forcing interactions with others, pretending to be interested, and exaggerating expressions or excitement.

> ### Note
> The term 'masking' is often used instead of 'camouflaging'; however, in clinical terms, masking is one of 3 aspects of camouflaging.

Camouflaging demands time, effort, and energy. Autistics often set aside time to rehearse social interactions, or to learn new social scripts from movies and books that they can use in real-life interactions. Acting and suppressing your true self takes a lot more energy and has significantly more consequences for your mental health than being authentic.[15, 16]

All this taken together, camouflaging can have a very negative impact on mental health, which increases the risk of getting into autistic burnout, or it can lead to autistic burnout faster. It can also increase how burned out you will become, and potentially even how long it will take to recover from it. For more information on camouflaging, search for the following four articles on our website:

Autism & camouflaging

AuDHD & camouflaging

Consequences of autistic camouflaging

Masking: is it good or bad?

3. Poor Mental Health

People struggling with mental health have more difficulty dealing with life stressors (i.e., the challenges of day-to-day living). Autistics in particular are more likely to experience anxiety, depression, PTSD, and sleep problems.[41, 42, 43]

1. **Anxiety:** Throughout life, **27–79%** of autistics experience clinical anxiety.[44, 45, 46] Anxiety disorders are diagnosed in **20%** of autistic adults compared to just **8.7%** of non-autistics.[42]

   → Anxiety in autistics is further increased by alexithymia; higher levels of alexithymia tends to lead to higher levels of anxiety.[47]

2. **Depression:** Between **37–48.6%** of autistics experience depression during their lifetime; and **25.9%** of autistics currently experience depression—compared to just **5%** of non-autistics.[44, 48, 49]

   → Up to **83.3%** of autistic children and adolescents experience depression.[50]

3. **PTSD:** Between **44–60%** of autistic adults experience PTSD at some time in their lives, compared to an estimated **5.6%** for the general population.[51]

4. **Sleep Disturbances:** Autistics experience much more sleep problems; research shows that **64.7–73%** of autistics are affected by them. Problems include taking longer to fall asleep, less continuous sleep, and waking up more in the middle of the night.[41]

   → Poor sleep is linked to a lower quality of life, which impacts day-to-day functioning of autistic people.[52] In other words, the worse the sleep, the worse the performance throughout the day.

   → For more information on the consequences of sleep problems in autism, have a look at the 'Effects' article of our autism & sleep problems series:

   Autism & sleep problems: Effects

5. **Other Psychiatric Conditions:** Autistics are more likely to experience psychiatric conditions; nearly **70%** of autistic children and adolescents experience at least one other condition alongside autism, and almost **40%** experience two or more.[53, 54]

   → Having more than one psychiatric condition can have a negative influence on the mental health factors mentioned above.

4. Executive Functioning Challenges

Many if not most autistics experience difficulties with executive functioning such as planning, organization, time management, flexibility, etc.[54] Autistics who struggle with executive functioning are less protected from autistic burnout.

For instance, those with low flexibility have difficulty with change and struggle to cope with daily stressors; and they find it harder to manage time and complete tasks. This can make seemingly simple tasks feel impossible. This increases the risk of getting into autistic burnout, and can make it more difficult to recover from it as well.

Those who have ADHD as well tend to experience more executive challenges, and will experience more of the consequences. This will apply to the majority of autistic people, as research shows that around **50–70%** of autistics have ADHD as well.[56]

5. Other

There are also risks that reduce your ability to manage demands, which can increase the chance of developing or worsening burnout.

These risks include:

1. **A greater number of autistic traits**
   - → More autistic traits means more difficulty in meeting demands that people and society place on you.[5]

2. **Sensory sensitivities**
   - → Sensory sensitivities make it more challenging to manage life demands, because you spend a lot of energy on managing and trying to prevent sensory overload.[56, 5, 2]

3. **A history of bullying, rejection, and trauma**
   - → Autistics experience more bullying and trauma than non-autistics. These experiences tend to result in poorer mental health.[58, 59]

4. **Low cognitive empathy**
   - → Being less able to draw conclusions about others' beliefs and knowledge reduces your general well-being, because you are less able to anticipate other people and respond appropriately.[60] This can have

a negative influence on you; when you're unable to perform as well as others in social situations or in the work environment, you are more likely to be excluded by others because of it.

5. Tendency for people-pleasing

→ Trying to keep others happy takes a lot of energy and effort. People-pleasing refers to focusing more on keeping others happy, even though this is a drain on you. It is an example of camouflaging, and can be seen as a 'fawn' trauma response. This is a response just like fight, flight, or freeze; except fawning has to do with people-pleasing, avoiding conflict, and doing everything you can not to anger or upset others. Autistics may use it as a way to protect themselves from becoming a victim, but people-pleasing can be dangerous in its own right.[61]

6. A tendency to experience shame, judge yourself, and have a low sense of self-worth

→ Autistics are more likely to see themselves in a negative way because of difficulties in social communication, and discrimination. These factors have a negative influence on your general mental health and your perceived sense of self-worth.[62, 63]

7. Having multiple marginalized identities (e.g., race, gender, sexuality, socioeconomic status, etc.)

→ Your intersectional identity relates to how much systemic oppression you experience. The more marginalized you are, the more discrimination you face. This impacts your mental health, how much effort you may put into trying to fit in, and ultimately contributes to your risk of experiencing burnout.

The risk of autistic burnout decreases when autistic people live as their authentic self, without the need to mask, and when they receive proper support and have their needs met. To achieve this, they have to accept and embrace their autistic traits, and learn to identify and meet their (support) needs.

Protective Factors

Factors that protect autistic people from autistic burnout include:[57, 5, 2]

- **'Stimming':** engaging in activities like fidgeting, rocking, spinning, rubbing fabric, or other ways to stimulate or self-soothe.

- **'Special interests':** partaking in their passions and interests.

- **Self-awareness**: being aware of signals inside the body (called 'interoception'), such as hunger, tiredness, or the need to use the bathroom. Self-awareness also includes being able to recognize the things that trigger you, so you can better prevent them or more swiftly process them when you do get triggered.

- **Self-efficacy:** taking care of yourself, focusing on your mental health, and setting and protecting your boundaries.

- **Social support:** family, friends, and the autistic community; basically any people you can rely on for support.

- **Access to accommodations:** adjustments to your school or work environment, such as extra time on tests, flexible work hours, or written instructions in addition to verbal ones, and healthcare that considers autistic-specific needs.

Special Cases

In this section, we look at the factors mentioned above from the perspective of several vulnerable groups.

1. Children and Teenagers

Parents, teachers, and medical professionals have to stay on the lookout for signs of burnout; autistic children and teenagers tend to be more devoted to their passions and are less likely than neurotypicals to ask for help on their own.[64]

In addition, they may struggle with self-awareness and alexithymia, which can make it more challenging for them to recognize a need for support.

Autistic children/teenagers are more likely to experience autistic burnout if they:

- Spend years in school camouflaging and masking.
- Go to school five days a week
- Often experience sensory sensitivities and social challenges at school and in after-school programs and activities
- Go to schools that don't offer as much support, especially support based on the particular needs of autistic children/teenagers
- Experience changes during puberty

2. Young Adults

Autistic burnout can lead to dropping out of university or periods of unemployment in young adults. This can cause setbacks for autistic people compared to others, both in finding a job again and earning a livable wage.

Recognizing increased risks is important for having ongoing support and accommodations in place for the future.

Some examples of situations that could put young autistic adults at a greater risk of autistic burnout are:

- Spending years in college or work camouflaging or masking
- Going to college or working full-time
- A lack of school or workplace accommodations, or not enough accommodations to learn or work comfortably
- Experiencing new sensory and social challenges at school or at work
- Moving away from home for the first time
- Managing daily tasks for the first time
- Living with unsupportive roommates in college dorms

3. Periods of Hormones Going Up and Down in Adulthood

Experiencing upcoming menopause symptoms in adults

Changes in hormone levels can have a negative influence on your thinking, emotions, and overall mental health, which can increase the risk of autistic burnout.[65]

This can be due to:

- Difficulty in changing behaviours based on the demands of your environment and social situations
- Unpredictable/big/new changes in mood/behaviour/body
- Changes in mental health due to depression and anxiety

Individuals who just gave birth to their child

In the weeks after giving birth (the 'postpartum' period), postpartum autistics are more likely to become burned out due to changes to mood and their ability to deal with executive challenges. The meaningful life change of caring for a new child can be overwhelming and cause major changes in their routine.

Diagnosing Autistic Burnout

Currently, there are no medical tests such as blood tests or brain scans that definitively diagnose autistic burnout. However, researchers have established the following provisional criteria for autistic burnout:[57]

The following symptoms must have been present for a period of at least **3** months, and represent a change from previous functioning:

1. **Significant mental and physical exhaustion.** An overwhelming sense of exhaustion is central to autistic burnout. It goes beyond ordinary tiredness, and significantly impacts physical and emotional well-being.

2. **Social withdrawal and reduced social engagement.** Burnout often leads to increased social withdrawal. Autistics may find it more challenging to engage in social contact during this period—choosing solitude as a means of coping.

3. **One or more of the following:**
   a. Significant reduced functioning in various areas (e.g., social, occupational, educational).
   b. Confusion, difficulties with executive function, and/or dissociative states.
   c. Increased autistic traits and/or a reduced capacity to camouflage/mask autistic characteristics and/or reduced tolerance of stimuli.

Autistic burnout may manifest as:[57]

- Increased emotional sensitivity, leading to being easily overwhelmed and experiencing more meltdowns or shutdowns.

- Changes in executive functioning, making it harder to plan and make decisions and cope with unexpected changes and disruptions in routine.

- Greater physical and mental exhaustion, resulting in an increased need for sleep and difficulty concentrating, completing tasks, remembering information, and keeping up with social demands.

> **Note**
>
> The infographic of the provisional criteria of autistic burnout on the following two pages will also come with this book as two separate files for easy printing; one with a horizontal layout (as shown), and one with a vertical layout.

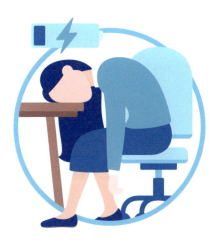

Diagnostic Criteria for Autistic Burnout

Autistic burnout is characterized by:

1 Significant Exhaustion

2 Increased Social Withdrawal

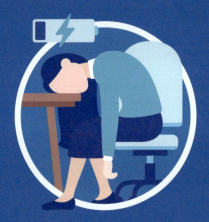

+

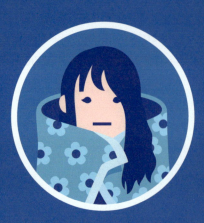

3 Plus one or more of the following:

Ⓐ Reduction in Functioning

Ⓑ More Executive Challenges

Ⓒ Reduced Capacity to Camouflage

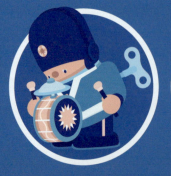

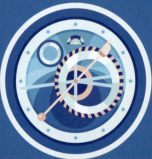

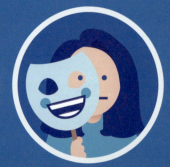

Provisional criteria for autistic burnout according to Higgins et al. (2021).

Autistic burnout can look like:

Greater Emotionality

→ Feeling more emotional
→ Prone to getting overwhelmed
→ Difficulty regulating emotions
→ Experiencing more meltdowns
→ Experiencing more shutdowns

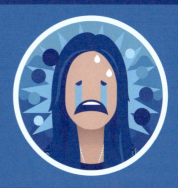

Executive Challenges

→ More difficulty planning things
→ More difficulty coping with unexpected changes
→ More difficulty coping with disruptions in routine
→ More difficulty making decisions

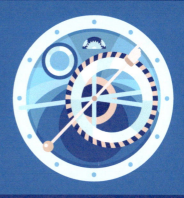

Significant Exhaustion

→ Feeling physically more exhausted
→ Feeling mentally more exhausted
→ Unable to think clearly
→ Difficulty concentrating
→ A harder time completing work
→ Difficulty remembering things
→ More need for rest
→ Unable to keep up with social demands

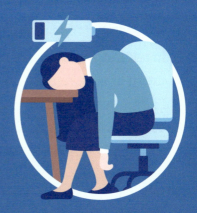

Common symptoms of autistic burnout according to Higgins et al. (2021).

What to Expect From Your Health Professional

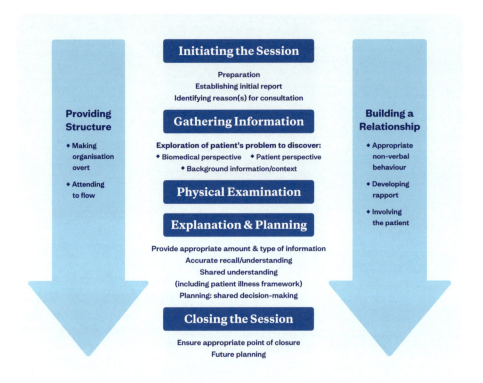

Providing Structure

Initiating the Session

Preparation
Establishing initial report
Identifying reason(s) for consultation

- Making organisation overt
- Attending to flow

Gathering Information

Exploration of patient's problem to discover:
- Biomedical perspective
- Patient perspective
- Background information/context

Physical Examination

Explanation & Planning

Provide appropriate amount & type of information
Accurate recall/understanding
Shared understanding
(including patient illness framework)
Planning: shared decision-making

Building a Relationship

- Appropriate non-verbal behaviour
- Developing rapport
- Involving the patient

Closing the Session

Ensure appropriate point of closure
Future planning

During a healthcare visit, healthcare professionals typically follow a specific script. Knowing this can help you maximize your time with your provider. Many autistics have challenges at healthcare visits because they do not know how to answer questions in a way that doctors are accustomed to.

In addition, doctors are trained to treat neurotypicals and do not get much or any training on the different ways an autistic may present. I have coached autistics about how to effectively communicate their condition to their health provider.

Before going to your appointment, it's helpful to prepare for the different phases of the visit.

A healthcare provider appointment generally consists of the following phases:

1. **Initiating the session**

   a. Greeting, which is usually in a non-autistic style. For example:

      i. "Hi, how are you?" (If the doctor or therapist has met you before.)

      ii. "Hello, I am Doctor X." (If the doctor has not met you before.)

2. **Gathering information**

   a. In a therapy session, the therapist tries to create rapport, so often the conversation will be more chatty. If the practitioner is chatty, it may not be clear for the autistic as to when they can discuss the purpose of their visit.

   b. Know that it is essential to say why you have come. As explained before, healthcare providers are not typically trained in autistic communication; however, they are indeed following a script. For example:

      i. They may ask a question about why you have come, such as:

         → What brings you here today?

         → How can I help you?

         → How are you doing?

      ii. They may ask questions from a symptom form (see the **Symptom Form** in the upcoming **Healthcare Visit** section).

3. **Examinations**
   a. The health professional may ask you to complete psychometric tests, where you will be given an often multiple-choice style quiz about your experience.
   b. The health professional may perform a physical examination, which may include visually examining, touching, and manipulating the area of concern.
4. **Assessing and diagnosing from the information gathered**
   a. They will provide an opinion about what the next step is. Some possible next steps may be:
      i.   Specialized tests that need a referral
      ii. Diagnosis and treatment protocol
      iii. Referral to a specialist
5. **Explanation to the patient**
   a. The health professional will ask if the patient has any questions about the doctor's opinion.
6. **Ending the session**
   a. Planning for a follow-up.
   b. Non-autistic ending of the session, such as:
      → "Have a good day."

Being aware of these phases can help you navigate the healthcare visit more effectively and ensure that your needs are effectively communicated and addressed.

Healthcare Visit

Preparing for your Healthcare Visit

Before going to your appointment, fill out a symptom form to describe your symptoms (find our **Symptom Sheet** in the **Patient Handouts** section at p. 218). Use one form/sheet per symptom—making it easier for your healthcare practitioner to process the information.

As an example, on the next page is the form Natalie filled out prior to her recent appointment regarding exhaustion:

Note

The severity of a symptom is probably the most difficult thing for an autistic person to describe, and they tend to underreport the severity. Consequently this leads to the healthcare practitioner not understanding the severity of the symptom—and even the seriousness of the situation.

It is best to describe how it is affecting your life, and it may be helpful to use the **Severity scale** (p. 219). Tell your medical practitioner both the description and number of the severity scale to properly inform them about the extent and impact.

Symptom Form for Medical Visit

Patient information	
Name:	Natalie E.
Age:	54
General description	
Symptom:	Very tired all the time
Where do you notice the symptom?	My whole body is tired.
Is it constant or intermittent? If intermittent, then when?	It has been constant, but it is unmanageable if I work more than 3 days a week.
How long does it last when it happens?	It has not stopped since Christmas.
Does it radiate anywhere (does it extend beyond the main area)?	No.
What other symptoms do you have with it?	I get nauseous when I work for too long. My eyes are always dry and burning. I also have developed pain on the right side of the base of my skull.

Severity of symptom	
Severity rating:	7; it's interfering with my day-to-day life.
What is the symptom interfering with in your life?	It has stopped me from taking my chess lessons and practicing chess. I am unable to clean the house and have asked someone to help me once a week for a bit. I also have someone to help me make meals once per week so that I have them and don't have to cook. People helping me is nice, but it also adds to my social contact.
Evolution of symptoms	
When did the symptom start?	I have been more tired than usual for quite a long time now, but this is different from my normal tiredness. This extreme tiredness started at Christmas time.
What was different in your life (in the month) before the symptom started?	Before Christmas, I had a busy schedule with more social contact. Unfortunately, my son and I got Covid during the holiday. I had to take care of my son and my 21-year-old dog while I was sick. After Christmas, I returned to work without fully recovering, and I had to take a break in February because I was so tired.
Has the symptom been getting better or worse?	It has been pretty bad all along and is only a little better if I severely limit my life.
How quickly has the symptom been getting better or worse?	It has not gotten better or worse; it has just stayed consistently bad.

Explored treatments	
What makes the symptom better or worse (e.g., food, sleep, stress)?	It is better when I avoid doing any activities. It is worse when I do more activities.
Medications?	Nothing.
Supplements?	Quercetin.
Physical therapy?	None.
Did any of the treatments help? If yes, how?	The Quercetin did not have any noticeable effect. Other treatments have not been explored.

Initiating the Session

Most healthcare providers will initiate the session with:

"Hello, I am Dr. A. What brings you here today?"

The doctor asks this question to understand which symptoms you would like to discuss.

Natalie:

To continue my example from earlier, when I saw a new doctor, the first thing I mentioned was that I am autistic. This served two purposes:

1. It informed me of how autism-aware the doctor was.
2. It lets the doctor know that I am autistic, which can be relevant to their medical considerations and treatment protocols.

I also always provide information that is important to know about myself:

1. I have **Mast Cell Activation Syndrome** (MCAS).

2. Due to being autistic, I need clear instructions.

> **Note**
>
> Effective communication is crucial in every doctor-patient interaction.

The Triple Empathy Problem

The **triple empathy problem**—which speaks to the challenges in neurotypical to autistic communication in healthcare settings—has recently been identified.[24]

Not only is it difficult for us to understand non-autistic communication, and difficult for non-autistics to understand us (captured by the **double empathy problem**[21] and the **dialectical misattunement hypothesis**);[22] but healthcare professionals often use complex medical terminology that is difficult to understand (called 'medical jargon').

Therefore, it's essential to ensure that your healthcare provider understands autism and its physiological differences, and that they are able to communicate to you in a way that you can understand.

On the next page is an example of communication between an autistic person and their medical practitioner going wrong due to this interpersonal mismatch of cognitive and communication styles.

An autistic female, age 15:

> An autistic went to their doctor to discuss their anxiety. They stated that going to the doctor in the first place was anxiety-inducing, and due to their severe daily anxiety, they were spending more time having panic attacks than not. Their doctor dismissed them and told the autistic patient that they did not have anxiety. The autistic responded with 'okay'.
>
> After the interaction, the autistic patient—feeling overpowered by the doctor's authority—ended up doubting their own experience of anxiety, preventing them from further pursuing the care and support they needed.

This highlights the need for a better understanding and communication between doctors (or medical practitioners in general) and autistics.

Gathering Information
History of Symptoms

When you visit your doctor, the first step is usually gathering information. Your doctor will ask you about the reason for your visit.

If possible, it may be helpful to fill out the **Symptom Sheet** found in the **Patient Handouts** section of this booklet (p. 218). Use one form for each symptom and reference the example I gave previously.

Since autistic burnout is linked to high suicide rates, the doctor will likely screen for suicide risk first. After ensuring that you are not at risk of harming yourself, the doctor will conduct a clinical interview. This interview involves a face-to-face verbal and nonverbal exchange between the clinician and the patient designed to gather the necessary data for diagnosis and treatment.

Psychometrics or Quizzes

Your doctor may use psychometrics or quizzes to evaluate if you are experiencing autistic burnout.

If you haven't been assessed for autism, your doctor might screen you for autism by giving you the **Autism Spectrum Quotient** (AQ) or the **RAADS–R** quiz. You might be asked to take the test at home.

If you've already been diagnosed, your doctor could administer the **Autistic Burnout Construct** (8 questions) or the **Copenhagen Burnout Inventory** (19 items; or 8 for just the personal burnout subscale).

Physical Exam

Your doctor may do a physical exam and order bloodwork based on the conversation they have with you.

Closing the Session

The doctor will end the session by informing you of when they need to see you again.

Clinical Approach

When working with individuals with autistic burnout. The following flow chart outlines the optimal course of action:

1. **Screen for suicide risk**
2. **Diagnose and determine cause and severity of autistic burnout**
   a. Conduct a clinical interview
      i. Collect a thorough history
      ii. Assess for environmental factors
      iii. Assess for risk factors

b. Administer psychometrics.

c. Diagnose based on current understanding
of diagnostic criteria.

3. **Treat autistic burnout**

a. Achieve remission of autistic burnout symptoms.

b. Restore optimal functioning.

c. Prevent relapse/recurrence.

Communication Guidelines for Medical Professionals

Autistics have different needs when it comes to communication than non-autistics, so it may be useful to discuss the following guidelines with your medical professional:

1. **Avoid social chit chat.** This is unnecessary to connect and develop a relationship and it often causes distress, anxiety, and overwhelm.

2. **Avoid assumptions based on nonverbal cues.** Autistic body language differs from non-autistic communication norms, and should not be used to gather information, as the healthcare provider could risk misinterpreting autistic nonverbal communication. They may unintentionally read into behaviours that were never meant to convey information. Examples of typical nonverbal communication styles in autistics:

   → "Unusual" eye contact or no eye contact.

   → Less pronounced facial expressions or a lack of facial expressions (called 'flat affect').

   → Less variations in tone of voice.

3. **Be careful not to confuse response styles with disinterest/resistance.** Autistics often do not follow expected social norms in communication. Take what they say at face value, and do not read too much into how it is said. Ask for clarity if there is uncertainty. For instance, sounding aloof does not indicate disinterest or a lack of motivation.

4. **Communicate with clarity.** Autistics are typically very literal. It is necessary to communicate directly (this is not "rude" or "insensitive"!) and avoid expressions or words that can be interpreted in different ways. Do not assume there is any subtext to what is being said, and avoid speaking with subtext yourself. The following can make communication more clear for autistic people:

   → Asking specific instead of open-ended questions.

   → Asking directly about the topic you are interested in. You cannot expect autistics to "know where you are going" with your questions

   → Explaining the purpose before asking a question instead of assuming you are both on the same page

5. **Give time for responses.** Autistics may take more time than non-autistics to process questions and come up with a response. To ensure the information you get will be accurate, autistics should not feel pressured to respond immediately. The following will aid in that:

   → Sharing questions/discussion topics ahead of your meeting

   → Allowing autistics to follow up with more information after the meeting

6. **Ask about communication needs.** Respect that many autistics know more about their communication needs than you do; so ask them about their particular needs. For example:

   → "Is there anything about the way you communicate that would be helpful for me to understand?"

   → "Is there anything that you need from me to make sure that communication between us goes smoothly?"

These guidelines were developed based on the lived experiences of autistics, and the Wales Autism Research Centre at Cardiff University.[65]

> **Note**
>
> Every autistic will differ in their communication needs. The best practice is to ask about theirs!

1. Screen for Suicide Risk

When someone with autism is exhausted, overwhelmed, depressed, or anxious, there is a higher risk of suicide.

Suicidality is a real risk for autistic individuals. About three-quarters of autistic individuals report having suicidal thoughts, and about half report attempting suicide.[67] Autistic individuals are **25** times more likely to attempt suicide compared to those without autism.[68]

Your clinician can administer the **Ask Suicide-Screening Questionnaire** (ASQ), which is an evidence-based suicide screening tool developed by the National Institute of Mental Health.[69] It takes less than one minute to administer.

2. Diagnose and Determine the Severity of Autistic Burnout

To fully understand an individual's condition and the extent of their autistic burnout, the healthcare provider should conduct a clinical interview, administer psychometric tests, and compare the presentation with the diagnostic criteria.

Clinical Interview

Your health care provider should conduct a thorough interview to determine the following:

1. Symptoms
2. How long you have had these symptoms
3. Your previous episodes of autistic burnout, if you have had any
4. How your symptoms are affecting your ability to work, socialize, etc.
5. What things worsen symptoms
6. What things lessen your symptoms
7. Co-occurring conditions, such as depression, anxiety disorders, and occupational burnout

Note that there is a high degree of overlap and misdiagnosis of depression and autistic burnout, so individuals who present with depression or suicidality should be screened for autistic burnout. Additionally, the healthcare provider should be sure to rule out physical causes, such as **long COVID, cardiovascular disease, thyroid conditions, chronic fatigue, dysautonomia,** and **Postural Orthostatic Tachycardia Syndrome** (POTS), as these are common comorbidities with autism.

Psychometrics

The following screening questions and assessment tools are recommended when autistic burnout is suspected:

Psychometrics for Autistic Burnout

Autistic Burnout Construct (ABO):[70] A self-assessment tool consisting of 8 questions measuring the *Exhaustion* dimension of autistic burnout.

☞ Embrace-Autism.com/Autistic-Burnout-Construct

Copenhagen Burnout Inventory (CBI):[71] A self-report measure consisting of 19 items, which measures three types of burnout: personal burnout, work-related burnout, and client-related burnout.

The 8-item *Personal Burnout* subscale measures autistic burnout,[4] but we found it useful to take the complete CBI to get a sense of how different factors and imposed demands contribute to your burnout.

☞ Embrace-Autism.com/Copenhagen-Burnout-Inventory

Psychometrics for Autism

Embrace Autism has a wide range of automated psychometrics to screen for autism, including:

Ritvo Autism Asperger Diagnostic Scale–Revised (RAADS–R):[72] A self-report designed to identify adult autistics who "escape diagnosis" due to having subtle traits that healthcare professionals may miss.

☞ Embrace-Autism.com/RAADS-R

The Autism Spectrum Quotient (AQ):[73] This is a highly validated, self-administered questionnaire that is used to measure autistic traits in adults.

☞ Embrace-Autism.com/Autism-Spectrum-Quotient

For more psychometrics to screen for autism and associated conditions (**ADHD, alexithymia, camouflaging/masking, trauma/PTSD,** etc.), have a look at Embrace Autism's 'Autism tests' page:

Embrace-Autism.com/autism-tests

Psychometrics for Depression

Beck Depression Inventory-II (BD-II):[74] This questionnaire measures traits of depression. Because **98%** of autistics with autistic burnout meet the threshold for a depression diagnosis, an assessment for depression is recommended when burnout is suspected.[4]

Psychometrics for Occupational Burnout

Copenhagen Burnout Inventory (CBI):[71] This self-assessment tool measures three types of burnout: personal burnout, work-related burnout, and client-related burnout. Use the *Work-related Burnout* subscale to measure occupational burnout specifically.

☞ Embrace-Autism.com/Copenhagen-Burnout-Inventory

Maslach Burnout Inventory™ (MBI):[75] This psychometric test is used to screen for occupational burnout, which can co-occur with and exacerbate autistic burnout.

3. Treating Autistic Burnout

In this section, we share treatments for autistic burnout that are suitable for autistic people.

Treatment Procedure

> ### Note
>
> These following steps may be difficult for autistics, especially for those with low self-awareness, alexithymia, and challenges in noticing the body's internal states. You may need support. Recognizing the signs of burnout is the initial step toward addressing and preventing it.

Beginning: Determine Suicide Risk

Use the **ASQ** (see also the **Screen for Suicide Risk** section at p. 150).

Step 1: Identify

Identify the life situations that put a lot of demands on you (see the **Causes** section at p. 106 for an extensive list). Fill out the **Energy Inventory** (p. 221) to get a sense of what drains you.

- **Demands:** Social demands, sensory demands, cognitive demands, and daily life demands

- **Changes**, such as life transitions

- **Parenting and relations.** For example, single parent or child-rearing conflicts, differing neurotypes where one person is autistic and the other is neurotypical

- **Employment**, including full-time work, in-person work, social interaction at work, autism awareness at work, and the commute

- **School environments**, including with a lack of accommodations or full-time studies
- **Co-occurrences:** ADHD, MCAS, POTS

Step 2: Retreat

- Ask for medical leave if possible
  - → The duration needed will depend on the severity and length of autistic burnout
  - → Reassess autistic burnout score every two months using the **ABO** or **CBI**

- **Request accommodations.** For example:
  - → Part-time hours
  - → Work from home
  - → Sensory accommodations

- **Withdraw from demands** (you can use the **Energy Inventory** (p. 221) to identify things that feel too demanding/draining)
  - → Be practical and realistic
  - → Inform people that withdrawal is not personal

- Prognosis
  - → Reacting to identify and address causes is the best prevention strategy
  - → If severe, recovering from burnout can take months or even years

Step 3: Restructure

- Environmental change is necessary, as it is often the source of autistic burnout.

- Consult an experienced autistic therapist, well-informed about autistic burnout. They can suggest ways to avoid or accommodate high levels of stress.

- Consider seeking disability leave for time to recuperate

- To prevent the return of autistic burnout, you must eliminate the conditions that caused it.

- Identify support needs to create accommodations.

Seek support:

- **Consider ways to communicate your needs to others**
  - → Explain daily challenges using speech, text, email, etc.
  - → Ask for help from friends and loved ones
  - → If safe, speak to human resources at work or a disability coordinator at school

- **Connect with others in the autistic community**
  - → Join a social support network online
  - → Look for others on social media; for instance, by searching and using hashtags like **#ActuallyAutistic**
  - → Seek out an autistic mentor

Step 4: Re-energize

- List the activities that re-energize you, and engage in them

- Engage in special interests during recovery (energy permitting). Create a plan for continued engagement before the next step

Step 5: Return and Reintegrate

Begin this step only when the **ABO** and/or **CBI–P** scores are **31** and **49** or lower, or when scored significantly lower than the initial score(s).

Gradual Return:

- Facilitation
    - → Reintegrate with the external world gradually.
    - → Return to daily activities and routines at a reduced level.
    - → Begin with half of what you believe you can do.
    - → Monitor for signs according to **Identify** (p. 154), and return to the step **Retreat** (p. 155) at the earliest signs of burnout.

> ### Note
> Additional adjustments might be needed to stabilize reintegration. Reintegration can be a recurring process if significant change and social support are required. It can be challenging to identify needs and accept limitations.

Drop the Mask

Masking and camouflaging can contribute to autistic burnout, as it not only takes a significant amount of effort and energy, but it can lead to cultivating a false persona, which undermines authentic and deep connections; it doesn't feel nice to be liked for who you present, rather than who you truly are. So being selective in when to employ this coping strategy is crucial for recovery and prevention.

- Where masking and camouflaging occur, make deliberate choices about their benefit or harm
- Prioritize authenticity

Masking and camouflaging are strategies that can help individuals stay safe in uncertain environments. This is especially important for autistic individuals with multiple marginalized identities, such as queer-trans and BIPOC autistics.

In some situations, it may not be safe or feasible to reveal one's true self. Therefore, a more realistic and practical approach could be to use masking in moderation.

The concept of safety, self-protection, and masking also applies to therapeutic settings. Masking and camouflaging behaviours can create obstacles to receiving the support needed.

When is Psychotherapy/Counselling Appropriate?

Psychological therapies need to be adapted to be effective for autistics. Therapists must understand the traits and needs of autistic people, and should not make assumptions based solely on the diagnosis of autism.[76] Question your assumptions and confirm them with your client.

> ### Note
> The goal of therapy should not be
> to decrease autism symptoms;
> only address what causes distress.[77]

Some examples of adaptations and accommodations:

- Virtual therapy is more comfortable and is equally as helpful for autistic adults; it reduces many barriers to obtaining healthcare; there is no need to travel or interact with staff and crowded waiting rooms; and it can be a sensory-friendly setting.

- Remove sensory stressors such as bright lights and loud ambient noises

- Make appointments routine so that the date, time, and place are predictable

- Request a communication style with direct questions, a consistent tone of voice, and no expectation of eye contact

- Reduce uncertainty with an agenda before each session

With appropriate adaptations in place, therapy can help support autistics with mental health challenges. Such support is crucial for preventing autistic burnout (see **Risk Factors** at p. 123).

Pharmacological Treatments

Autistic burnout does not require medication. Its causes are attributed to external factors rather than internal physiological differences.[78] Medications such as Selective Serotonin Reuptake Inhibitors (SSRIs) may help treat autistic burnout by indirectly supporting co-occurring conditions such as depression and anxiety.

It is important to note that studies have used medications to target core features of autism rather than focusing on mental health conditions in autistic people. Autistic traits should not be seen as needing to be "cured" or "reduced." Using medications in this manner can stigmatize autistics as abnormal.

Co-occurrences

Autistic burnout commonly occurs alongside:

- **Depression**
  - → **98%** of autistics with autistic burnout have **Major Depressive Disorder.**[79] Autistic people are four times more likely to develop depression than the general population. It is even considered the most common mental health condition in autistic people.

- **Occupational burnout**
  - → A 2022 study found that the prevalence of occupational burnout in the general population ranged from **19–38%.**[80] These statistics apply to autistic people as well; and given that there is some overlap between occupational and autistic burnout in terms of imposed demands and lack of support to deal with those demands, autistic people may be particularly susceptible to occupational burnout.[81, 42, 43, 82]

  - → A 2023 study cite that risk factors for occupational burnout were (**1**) being female, (**2**) having a lower quality of life, (**3**) experiencing chronic pain, (**4**) mental health struggles, and (**5**) sleep disturbance.[83] These are common lived experiences in the autistic population, which again suggests that autistics are more susceptible to occupational burnout than the general population.

- **Attention Deficit Hyperactivity Disorder (ADHD)**
  - → Research shows that around **50–70%** of autistics also have ADHD (the co-occurrence is colloquially referred to as **AuDHD**).[56] Similar to autistic traits, ADHD traits may become more noticeable during burnout.

- **Alexithymia**
  - → Alexithymia is incredibly common among autistics. Research indicates that at least **49.93%** of autistics have alexithymia, with some studies suggesting the prevalence to be as high as **85%** for those experiencing mild to severe alexithymia—compared to a range of **4.89–13%** in the general population.[37, 38, 39, 40]
  - → This prevalence is highly significant, as some features commonly associated with autism are actually attributed to alexithymia rather than autism itself.
- **Autoimmune conditions**
  - → Several studies have shown an increased prevalence of autoimmune diseases such as **type 1 diabetes, rheumatoid arthritis** (RA), **hypothyroidism** due to **Hashimoto's disease, psoriasis,** and **systemic lupus erythematosus** among first-degree relatives of autistic individuals.[84, 85]
- **Post-traumatic stress disorder (PTSD)**
  - → A traumatic event usually causes PTSD. Individuals with PTSD may experience flashbacks or nightmares related to the traumatic event, which is not the case for autistic people without PTSD.
  - → About **44–60%** of autistic adults experience PTSD at some point in their life,[86, 87] compared to just **5.6%** of the general population.[51]

Characterizing Autistic Burnout

Autistic burnout results from chronic life stress, the conflict of demands versus abilities, and limited support. Its signs are exhaustion, cognitive changes, more noticeable autistic traits, and social withdrawal.

Signs of Autistic Burnout

The **ECAO** acronym describes signs of autistic burnout. Its basis is the **Autistic Burnout Severity Items** (ABSI).[79]

1. Exhaustion (E)

- Mental and physical exhaustion
- Social withdrawal
- A desire to do as little as possible
- Potential worsening of physical health
- Low self-esteem and self-efficacy
- Reliable coping methods are no longer helpful
- Previously enjoyable things are no longer enjoyable
- Dropping out of university or unemployment
- Signs of exhaustion that last for months to years

2. Cognitive Disruption (C), Memory Problems, Confusion, and Mood

- Decrease in functioning
  - → For example, reduced self-care, emotional imbalance, or selective mutism

- New executive functioning challenges
  - → For example, it may appear as though a person has traits of ADHD
- Reduction in cognitive processing
  - → For example, 'brain fog'
- Confusion about whether the signs are of clinical depression
  - → This confusion may be in the individual or in clinicians unfamiliar with autistic burnout
- Difficulty reporting emotional exhaustion and asking for help
- Decreased sense of personal accomplishment
- Overall worsening of mental health and changes in mood
  - → For example: despair, negativity, depression, irritability, and suicidality

3. Heightened Autistic Self-Awareness (A)

- Increased sensory sensitivity and self-awareness of autistic traits
- Increased display of autistic traits
  - → **Note:** Many autistic traits are considered coping mechanisms; their increase signifies an increase in engagement with coping techniques
- Decrease in camouflaging
  - → Camouflaging decreases because of capacity rather than choice
- Autistic burnout may come before and initiate an autism diagnosis
- Lower tolerance of sensory and social input

4. Overwhelm & Withdrawal (O)

- More shutdowns
  - → For example, being frozen—unable to do anything or move
  - → **Note:** Shutdowns can mimic burnout, but shutdowns are temporary. They last for minutes to days. Burnout is chronic and lasts from months to years
- Need for social withdrawal, recovery, and downtime
- Can include complete social isolation
  - → For example, hibernation, sleep
- Suicidal ideation, attempt, or completion
  - → Brought on by feelings of 'needing a way out'
  - → **44%** of autistics in burnout experience suicidality[57]

Differential Diagnoses

Autistic burnout can be misinterpreted as depression, occupational burnout, or chronic fatigue. This confusion can delay recovery and even worsen symptoms. Knowing how to distinguish the two is essential for autistics.

Depression vs. Autistic Burnout

> "Depression is the side effect, with burnout being the cause"
>
> **Participant in the research of Arnold et al. (2023)**

98% of autistics with autistic burnout surpass the cut-off for a depression diagnosis. Although this shows a significant overlap, burnout and depression have unique causes and conflicting treatments.[74] This summary shows how depression and autistic burnout compare.[74, 2]

Autistic Burnout	Depression
1. Behavioural change	
An apparent increase in autistic traits, such as sensory sensitivities, difficulty processing social and emotional information, and increased desire for repetition and sameness.	A change in mood, such as feeling low, despondent, and despair. Triad of maladaptive thinking. For example, thinking, "I am bad, the world is bad, and it is always going to be this way."
2. Passions and interests	
Engaging in 'special interests' is energizing.	Reduced enjoyment of passions and interests.
3. Social withdrawal	
Pervasive, and considered a coping mechanism; a recovery tool.	Social withdrawal can be a cause and furtherance of depression.
4. Somatic symptoms	
Increased fatigue potentially requiring more sleep to recover, but sleep disturbance is not a main feature.	Appetite and sleep disturbances; increased sleep does not promote recovery.

Occupational Burnout

Autistics with job-related burnout may show symptoms similar to someone with autistic burnout.[89] However, autistic burnout has various non-work-related causes. Limiting diagnoses to occupational burnout makes it harder for the autistic to get the support they need to recover and prevent the burnout from reoccurring.

Autistic burnout—but not occupational burnout—can be caused by the following:

- Social demands
- Sensory demands
- Demands of daily tasks
- Changes in routine and unexpected life events
- Insufficient support

Comparisons with Occupational Burnout

Autistic burnout is distinct from occupational burnout, with unique causes—and the potential for an individual to experience both.[2]

Autistic individuals are at a higher risk of burnout, which can result from long periods of general stress, extending beyond work relationships. This risk is much higher than the **25%** rate for occupational burnout in the general population.[2]

The rate of occupational burnout varies, with **25%** of workers reporting burnout overall. However, certain professions face higher rates, such as **50%** for postal workers,[83] **57%** for resident physicians,[90] and **24%** for physical education teachers.[91]

Several factors contribute to occupational burnout among postal workers—such as gender, quality of life, chronic pain, mental health issues, and sleep disturbances. These are also common factors in the autistic population, suggesting that autistic individuals are particularly vulnerable to burnout.

Chronic Fatigue Syndrome

Chronic fatigue syndrome (ME/CFS) and autistic burnout share some overlapping symptoms. Both conditions are characterized by severe exhaustion or fatigue and cognitive difficulties. Similar to

ME/CFS, autistic burnout symptoms can persist for years without proper diagnosis and intervention.[92]

However, the causes of ME/CFS and autistic burnout differ. Autistic burnout is closely related to prolonged stress, demands being beyond what they can do, and a lack of support related to disability. A comprehensive review of medical history and the identification of environmental stressors can help differentiate between the two conditions.[57]

Consequences of Autistic Burnout
Negative Impacts

Autistic burnout has negative consequences for mental and physical health. It affects employment capacity, independent living, overall quality of life, and well-being.[2]

Impacts on overall functioning include:[5]

- Exhaustion and an inability to function
- Decreased ability to produce and process speech
- Loss of previously acquired skills
- Heightened sensitivity to sensory input
- Reduced executive function

Impacts on mental health include:[79, 5]

- Suicidality
- Depression
- Anxiety

Possible secondary impacts of autistic burnout include:[2]

- Not achieving academic or employment potential
- Lack of self-fulfillment and personal potential
- Relationship difficulties
- Institutionalization
- Homelessness

Positive Impacts

Burnout can be the beginning of identity-awareness in undiagnosed autistics. Many are unaware that their struggles stem from trying to live a 'neurotypical life'.

When an undiagnosed autistic reaches a crisis point, seeking professional support from a medical professional may lead to:[2]

- A formal autism diagnosis
- Better self-awareness
- Improved self-care
- A new perspective on the past
- Increased self-worth
- Increased belief in personal abilities
- Avenues for community support
- Exploration of self-identity

Conclusion

Prevention and recovery are the priorities of treatment for autistic burnout.[5] For undiagnosed adults, seeking support can lead to self-discovery and an enhanced quality of life.

Autistic burnout is caused by the demands of living in a neurotypical society. Environmental factors, such as social, sensory, daily life, work, and cognitive demands exceed the capacity of many autistic individuals leading to or exacerbating autistic burnout. This is particularly true for individuals who have poor mental health, engage in masking or camouflaging, and have low self-awareness. Autistics in burnout experience exhaustion, cognitive and mood changes, a heightening of autistic traits (and a reduced ability to mask or camouflage), and withdrawal.

Autistics in burnout can recover by withdrawing and resting, identifying areas in their lives where changes are needed and support or accommodations are required, engaging in special interests, and gradually reintegrating into society.

Recovery is also facilitated by accessing social supports, spending time with fellow autistics, living more authentically (reducing camouflaging), and seeking therapy to improve self-awareness.

Footnotes

1. "Having All of Your Internal Resources Exhausted Beyond Measure and Being Left with No Clean-Up Crew": Defining Autistic Burnout (Raymaker et al., 2020)

2. Prevalence and Disparities in the Detection of Autism Without Intellectual Disability (Shenouda et al., 2023)

3. The experiences of autistic doctors: a cross-sectional study (Shaw et al., 2023)

4. Measuring and validating autistic burnout (Mantzalas et al., 2024)

5. A conceptual model of risk and protective factors for autistic burnout (Mantzalas et al., 2022)

6. Data and Statistics on Autism Spectrum Disorder: Prevalence of ASD (Centers for Disease Control and Prevention, 2023)

7. Autism spectrum disorder: Highlights from the 2019 Canadian health survey on children and youth (Public Health Agency of Canada, 2022)

8. Global prevalence of autism: A systematic review update (Zeidan et al., 2022)

9. Male to female ratios in autism spectrum disorders by age, intellectual disability and attention-deficit/hyperactivity disorder (Posserud et al., 2021)

10. What is the Male-to-Female Ratio in Autism Spectrum Disorder? A Systematic Review and Meta-Analysis (Loomes et al., 2017)

11. Finding the True Number of Females with Autistic Spectrum Disorder by Estimating the Biases in Initial Recognition and Clinical Diagnosis (McCrossin, 2022)

12. Community Reports on Autism 2023 (ADDM, 2023)

26. Reduced behavioral flexibility in autism spectrum disorders (D'Cruz et al., 2013)

27. The comorbidity between autism spectrum disorder and post-traumatic stress disorder is mediated by brooding rumination (Golan et al., 2021)

28. About Autism Spectrum Disorder (Centers for Disease Control and Prevention, n.d.)

29. The experiences of autistic doctors: a cross-sectional study (Shaw et al., 2023)

30. "I'm trying to reach out, I'm trying to find my people": A Mixed-Methods investigation of the link between sensory differences, loneliness, and mental health in autistic and nonautistic adults (Quadt et al., 2023)

31. Online Course: Autistic Burnout (Attwood and Garnett, 2024)

32. Workplace Discrimination against Individuals with Autism Spectrum Disorder (ASD) (Cooper & Mujtaba, 2022)

33. Policy on ableism and discrimination based on disability: Forms of discrimination (Ontario Human Rights Commission, n.d.)

34. A model for developing disability confidence (Lindsay & Canceliere, 2017)

35. Does volunteering with children affect attitudes toward adults with disabilities? A Prospective study of Unequal Contact (Fichten et al., 2005)

36. The Disability Employment Puzzle: A field experiment on employer hiring behavior (Ameri et al., 2017)

37. Investigating alexithymia in autism: A systematic review and meta-analysis (Kinnaird et al., 2019)

38. Measuring the effects of alexithymia on perception of emotional vocalizations in autistic spectrum disorder and typical development (Heaton et al., 2012)

39. Age is strongly associated with alexithymia in the general population (Mattila et al., 2006)

40. Prevalence of alexithymia and its association with sociodemographic variables in the general population of Finland (Salminen et al., 1999)

41. Sleep in adults with Autism Spectrum Disorder: A systematic review and meta-analysis of subjective and objective studies (Morgan et al., 2020)

42. Anxiety Disorders in Adults with Autism Spectrum Disorder: A Population-Based Study (Nimmo-Smith, et al., 2019)

43. Experience of trauma and PTSD symptoms in autistic adults: Risk of PTSD development following DSM-5 and Non-DSM-5 traumatic life events (Rumball et al., 2020)

44. Anxiety and depression in adults with autism spectrum disorder: a systematic review and meta-analysis (Hollocks et al., 2018)

45. Prevalence of Anxiety in Autism Spectrum Disorders (Kent & Simonoff, 2017)

46. A Scoping Review of Anxiety in Young Children with Autism Spectrum Disorder (Vasa et al., 2020)

47. Alexithymia in Adolescents with Autism Spectrum Disorder: Its Relationship to Internalising Difficulties, Sensory Modulation and Social Cognition (Milosavljevic et al., 2015)

48. Prevalence of Depressive Disorders in Individuals with Autism Spectrum Disorder: a Meta-Analysis. Journal of Abnormal Child Psychology (Hudson et al., 2019)

49. Depressive disorder (depression) (World Health Organization, 2023)

50. A systematic review of the rates of depression in autistic children and adolescents without intellectual disability (Stewart et al., 2021)

51. Trauma exposure and post-traumatic stress disorder in the general population (Frans et al., 2005)

52. Sleep determines quality of life in autistic adults: A longitudinal study (Deserno et al., 2019)

53. Prevalence of comorbid psychiatric disorders among people with autism spectrum disorder: An umbrella review of systematic reviews and meta-analyses (Hossain et al., 2020)

54. Depression in Children and Adolescents with Autism Spectrum Disorder (DeFilippis, 2018)

55. Executive Function in Autism Spectrum Disorder: History, Theoretical Models, Empirical Findings, and Potential as an Endophenotype (Demetriou et al., 2019)

56. The Prevalence of Attention Deficit/Hyperactivity Disorder Symptoms in Children and Adolescents With Autism Spectrum Disorder Without Intellectual Disability: A Systematic Review (Eaton et al., 2023)

57. Defining autistic burnout through experts by lived experience: Grounded Delphi method investigating #AutisticBurnout (Higgins et al., 2021)

58. Association of Autistic Traits With Depression From Childhood to Age 18 Years (Rai et al., 2018)

59. Association of autistic traits in adulthood with childhood abuse, interpersonal victimization, and posttraumatic stress (Roberts et al., 2015)

60. Cognitive empathy moderates the relationship between affective empathy and wellbeing in adolescents with autism spectrum disorder (Bos & Stokes, 2019)

61. 'I felt like I deserved it because I was autistic': Understanding the impact of interpersonal victimisation in the lives of autistic people (Pearson et al., 2022)

62. Social identity, self-esteem, and mental health in autism (Cooper et al., 2017)

63. How I See and Feel About Myself: Domain-Specific Self-Concept and Self-Esteem in Autistic Adults (Nguyen, et al., 2020)

64. Lower help-seeking intentions mediate subsequent depressive symptoms among adolescents with high autistic traits: A population-based cohort study (Hosozawa et al., 2023)

65. Cognition and mental health in menopause: A review (Hogervorst et al., 2021)

66. WARC's Guidelines for Interviewing Autistic Individuals (Winn, 2015)

67. A systematic review and meta-analysis of suicidality in autistic and possibly autistic people without co-occurring intellectual disability (Newell et al., 2023)

68. Recent Research Points to a Clear Conclusion: Autistic People are Thinking About, and Dying by, Suicide at High Rates (Conner, 2023)

69. Validation of the Ask Suicide-Screening Questions for adult medical inpatients: A brief tool for all ages (Horowitz et al., 2020)

70. The reliability and validity of a novel autistic burnout measure among neurodiverse college students (Richards et al., 2023)

71. The Copenhagen Burnout Inventory: A new tool for the assessment of burnout (Kristensen et al., 2005)

72. Ritvo Autism Asperger Diagnostic Scale–Revised (RAADS–R) (Ritvo et al., 2010)

73. The Autism-Spectrum Quotient (AQ): Evidence from Asperger Syndrome/High-Functioning Autism, Males and Females, Scientists and Mathematicians (Baron-Cohen, S., Wheelwright, S., Skinner, R. et al., 2001)

74. Beck Depression Inventory–II (BDI-II) (Beck et al., 1996)

75. Maslach Burnout Inventory manual (3rd ed.). (Masclack et al., 1996)

76. Using EMDR with autistic individuals: A Delphi survey with EMDR therapists (Fisher et al., 2023)

77. Neurodivergence-informed therapy (Chapman & Botha, 2023)

78. Benefits and harms of interventions to improve anxiety, depression, and other mental health outcomes for autistic people: A systematic review and network meta-analysis of randomised controlled trials (Linden et al., 2022)

79. Towards the measurement of autistic burnout (Arnold et al., 2023)

80. Addressing employee burnout: Are you solving the right problem? (McKinsey Health Institute, 2022)

81. A systematic review of quality of life of adults on the autism spectrum (Ayres et al., 2018)

82. National prevalence of pain among children and adolescents with autism spectrum disorders (Whitney & Shapiro, 2019)

83. The prevalence and risk factors of burnout and its association with mental issues and quality of life among Hungarian postal workers: a cross-sectional study (Kovács et al., 2023)

84. Comorbidity of allergic and autoimmune diseases in patients with autism spectrum disorder: A nationwide population-based study (Chen et al., 2013)

85. Maternal autoimmune diseases and the risk of autism spectrum disorders in offspring: A systematic review and meta-analysis (Chen et al., 2016)

86. Interpersonal trauma and posttraumatic stress in autistic adults (Reuben et al., 2021)

87. Experience of trauma and PTSD symptoms in autistic adults: Risk of PTSD development following DSM-5 and Non-DSM-5 traumatic life events (Rumball et al., 2020)

88. Trauma exposure and post-traumatic stress disorder in the general population (Frans et al., 2005)

89. "Psychology Works" Fact Sheet: Workplace Burnout (Canadian Psychology Association, 2021)

90. Prevalence of Occupational Burnout among Resident Doctors Working in Public Sector Hospitals in Mumbai (Dhusia et al., 2019)

91. Occupational burnout prevalence and its determinants among physical education teachers: A systematic review and meta-analysis (Alsalhe et al., 2021)

92. Myalgic Encephalomyelitis/Chronic Fatigue Syndrome. (Centers for Disease Control and Prevention, n.d.)

Autistic Burnout Stories

On the following pages are various accounts
of the lived experience of autistic burnout

Shana Aisenberg

Diagnoses:	**Autism, possible ADHD, alexithymia**
Age:	**68**
Diagnosed at:	**65 (self-diagnosed)**
Gender:	**Trans, non-binary, she/they**
Burnout type:	**Moderate**

I'm self-diagnosed autistic. I figured out that I was autistic around three years ago, in my mid-60s. I'd wondered about autism a few decades ago when getting to know someone who identified as Aspie; however, at the time, I didn't think I fit the criteria (which I'd taken very literally) and discounted it.

I'm a self-employed musician, composer, and music teacher, also working as a music director in a Unitarian Universalist church for the past nine years. Music has always been my passion and is, in many ways, my first language. I hear musical patterns and am nerdy about music theory. While work situations can sometimes be challenging, focusing on music also sustains me.

I'm in a state of burnout even as I write this. It's interesting to be writing about burnout from this perspective. I've been experiencing mild-to-moderate burnout for a few years; however, I didn't realize it for a while. As I've been in the process of unmasking, understanding various ways in which I'm overwhelmed by sensory experiences, and learning to recognize when I'm feeling dysregulated or when I'm in a state of meltdown or shutdown, I've been able to start figuring out how to manage burnout, how to make accommodations for myself.

Some ways in which burnout manifests for me: I'm finding it harder to keep my house clean, to declutter, to stay on top of replying to emails, to go through piles of paper, mail, etc., that have accumulated over the past few years. It can often be challenging to figure out what I want to eat or decide what to cook. Sensory issues around light and sound seem more pronounced. Although I can be hyperverbal (talking out loud is how I process things) when I'm dysregulated, it feels harder to speak—to find the words. In burnout, I become overwhelmed more easily, and get upset even by small things.

Some ways in which I'm managing burnout: I researched and recently got prescription rose-tinted FL-41 glasses, which are helping with light sensitivity. I've researched and bought earplugs to use when in noisy environments. I'm learning to say "no" to doing various things, even things I might typically enjoy doing, and I'm becoming more aware of how they might negatively impact me. I'm learning to recognize what I'm feeling; and I'm figuring out ways of stimming that help.

Most importantly, understanding my autism and burnout is helping me recognize when I feel overwhelmed, which—sometimes—allows me to change course before things get worse.

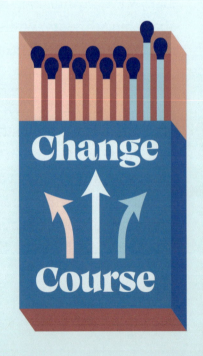

Allie Anderson

Diagnoses:	**Autism, ADHD, PDA, RSD**
Age:	**29**
Diagnosed at:	**28**
Gender:	**Female; she/her**
Burnout type:	**Severe**

Growing up, I knew I was different. I was a little girl with hard emotions who felt the world was against her. Since I brought others such joy while I felt so miserable, I convinced myself that I existed only for others. I put high pressure on myself for as long as I can remember, but I kept my struggles to myself.

The only "bad" they saw was the physical illnesses I couldn't control. I constantly had sinus infections and various illnesses, forcing me to miss school and eventually work. Oftentimes, I wouldn't even be sick, but I would use it as a way to lay in bed all day because I felt so anxious and dysregulated. Although I've experienced all levels of burnout throughout my life, this is my story of severe burnout.

I graduated with my MSW (Master of Social Work) in December of '21, and earned my professional licensure the next month. I was so excited to start my career in medical social work—I felt like I had finally found my place! I landed a renal social worker job with a large dialysis company. It was a lot of work and a lot of pressure. On the outside, I was thriving. I received accolades from my upper management, coworkers, and patients. On the inside, I was a total mess.

After months of trial and error in trying to figure out "why" I felt so bad, I came across multiple TikTok videos about autism and just about lost my mind. For the first time in my life, I had a name for everything I've been feeling, but surely I can't be autistic, right? Wrong! Once I acknowledged it was likely I had AuDHD, I couldn't unsee it.

My work performance stayed high, but it consumed my life. I avoided going to the clinic floor because I learned I was overstimulated, and the required amount of daily socialization was too much for me. However, I loved the idea of my job and knew I was making a difference despite my distress. I was constantly sick, I was avoiding my tasks at work for the first time, and I was feeling beyond hopeless. I was in tears on the way home nearly every day, spending hours after I got home curled up in a ball on the couch. Every day felt like too much, and yet I kept doing it.

One day, I woke up and couldn't get out of bed. I was terrified because I didn't understand, "Nothing is physically wrong, just stand up!" My body had finally had enough. I took a medical leave of absence for two months. I thought I could give my body that time to rest and be fine. However, I had to quit and have been unable to work as of writing this in '24. I recognized not only did I have burnout from work, but I also had severe autistic burnout that had been building up for honestly my whole life. So I talked to my partner and decided to take time off to heal and unmask, or I would be in a much worse position.

Slowly—over the next two years—I started to function more. I sought out a formal diagnosis to help better understand my autism, I joined group therapy for neurodivergent adults, and I worked on listening to what my own body was trying to tell me, rather than what I thought I was "supposed" to be feeling.

The process has been all-consuming and extremely difficult to explain to those around me. Autistic burnout is taking more time for me to work through than my job burnout, and that is OK. I'm proud of myself and the work I've done despite feeling like I didn't have a choice. I now believe that I can still be successful but also honor my unique needs with proper accommodations.

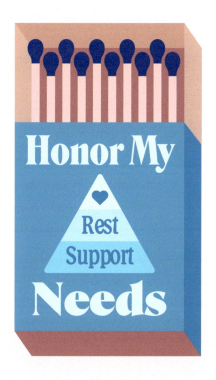

L. B.

Diagnoses:	**Autism, ADHD, alexithymia**
Age:	**48**
Diagnosed at:	**46**
Gender:	**Female; she/they**
Burnout type:	**Moderate**

The aftermath of the pandemic in my workplace and a change in management has made my workplace increasingly overstimulating and overwhelming.

I also volunteer at my spiritual center; and over time, I've ended up with increasingly heavy responsibilities at our periodic retreats, leaving me totally drained of energy and sometimes with limited ability to speak for days afterward because of the overwhelm.

The result is an overall trend of my becoming increasingly more sensitive to all stimuli, such as fluorescent lights, warm air, or chaotic auditory stimulation, such as multiple people speaking simultaneously. I now use grocery delivery services because stepping into grocery stores has become too overstimulating. I require multiple recovery days after any social activity, even those I enjoy. Some days, I can barely care for myself and must lie in bed most of the day.

I've reduced my work hours to 22 hours per week, which has helped somewhat but increased financial stress. I've requested work accommodations, though I continue to fight with HR to receive them after nine months, which has drained even more energy.

I've tried setting boundaries with my commitments at my spiritual center, though I've found that I am often not believed when I discuss my limitations. People seem not to understand why I used to be able to do certain tasks that I can no longer do.

One of the worst parts about autistic burnout is that despite undergoing a serious mental and physical health condition, it is invisible to most people around me.

It would help so much just to be heard and understood, and to have my energy limits respected by the people around me.

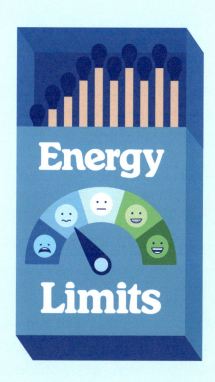

Carla Marina Costa

Diagnoses:	**Autism, ADHD**
Age:	**51**
Diagnosed at:	**51 (self-diagnosed)**
Gender:	**Female; she/her**
Burnout type:	**Severe**

I was 20 years old. I lived alone in Niteroi and studied and worked in Rio de Janeiro. I spent four to five hours daily on public transportation going from one place to another. It was during my graduation year as a science teacher, and I had a part-time job at a research institute at the university (UFRJ). I had a grueling routine and lost my voice the week before my first examination class. The doctor saw no problem with my vocal cords, and my voice returned the day before the second examination. My graduation memories are a blur; we received our certificate to register as teachers. But I was going to keep working at the institute.

I started to work in the institute full-time, and I had weekly headaches. Two months later, I went to a congress representing the institute with a panel of my work—a 51-hour bus journey from Rio to São Luis do Maranhão. I stayed there for a week and had relations with someone, which I only did it because I thought it was what I was supposed to do.

The next day, I had a headache that lasted for a week. From then on, every day was a struggle. I started smoking, and my job performance suffered. The weekends were the worst. I felt my heart heavy all the time. I couldn't sleep and moved through my day like an automaton. My headaches were constant, and the suicidal thoughts began.

I believe that my autism saved me from dying. The same day I contemplated jumping from a window was the day I decided to keep living one day at a time.

I left my job and went back home to start work as a teacher. I married two years later, had another burnout when my first child was born, and stopped working for good after the birth of my second son. I'm okay now.

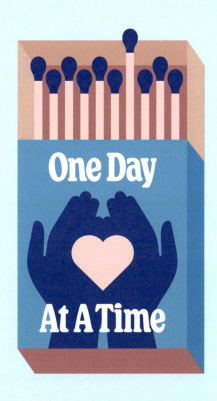

O. D.

Diagnoses:	**Autism, ADHD, cPTSD**
Age:	**32**
Diagnosed at:	**29**
Gender:	**Genderqueer; she/they**
Burnout type:	**Severe**

For me, autistic burnout was a slow buildup from years of masking, high expectations of achievement, and navigating neurotypical systems without knowing why they didn't work for me.

I began experiencing cyclical mild to moderate burnout in my teens. I was able to partially recover each time by reducing my output and responsibilities, but because I didn't know I was autistic, I lacked the information necessary to facilitate true recovery; I recovered just enough to be functional again, then returned to the same lifestyle and expectations that caused the burnout in the first place.

This chronic state of operating at a barely tolerable level meant that every time I burnt out, my functioning baseline continued to decrease. By the time I graduated from university, I was facing a near-constant private struggle with depression and anxiety. I dropped out of graduate school after one semester because I couldn't handle the workload anymore, and I worked full-time as an engineer for the next three and a half years. I cried on my way to work nearly every day and often hid in the bathroom with the lights off to get some respite from the sensory and social overwhelm of the office environment.

Eventually, I could no longer keep up with the burnout, and it continued to worsen without any degree of recovery. I isolated myself from my loved ones, my physical health deteriorated with increasingly frequent migraines and unexplained GI and cardiac issues, and my depression became dire. I quit my job out of necessity for my health, and the difficulties that continued in the subsequent few years ultimately led to my autism and ADHD diagnoses.

With this information and the help of a neurodivergence-focused therapist, I finally began to understand my needs, and rebuilt my health. I'm actively learning to accommodate myself in my daily life, listen to my nervous system, and set boundaries to protect myself from future burnout.

Due to skill regression, I still struggle with many aspects of life and gainful employment. However, I'm mentally healthier than ever, living independently, and I'm genuinely proud of how far I've come.

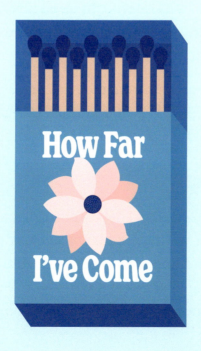

Stephanie H.

Diagnoses:	**Autism**
Age:	**52**
Diagnosed at:	**50**
Gender:	**Female; she/her**
Burnout type:	**Severe**

I am currently 53 years old and live in north central Florida. Since we moved around a lot, I grew up in many places. I lived in various cities in Florida, Virginia, and California.

I got my Master's in Education and taught the first six years at a Montessori school. Then, I taught in public school for 19 ½ years.

I had been very stressed at work the few years before my severe burnout. My teaching responsibilities had become overwhelming. The lockdown for COVID-19 brought on additional stress. I became the online technology teacher for the grade level. Every day, I taught 33 students over Zoom.

I decided I needed a break from the regular classroom. I moved to another school as the art teacher for the 2022–2023 school year—a school that did not have a comparable support system among the teachers. There were severe behavior issues I had to deal with from some of the students.

My health began declining. I developed a bleeding stomach ulcer and almost died. I went back for a while but quit after the first semester. My main symptoms of burnout were stress, developing an ulcer, having panic attacks on the way to work each day, headaches, sounds bothering me, and not being able to handle minor issues that I usually would be able to handle.

It took me a while to get over the burnout. Removing myself from that situation is what helped the most. I have a wonderful husband who convinced me it was time to quit. I am now working at a private school teaching third grade. My grandchildren all attend the same school, so I love that. The school environment is relaxed and wonderful.

To help prevent burnout in the future, I am very conscious of how much I do each day. I make sure not to do too much because that will exacerbate my health issues and make the stress worse. I enjoy life at home more and take time to have fun with my family.

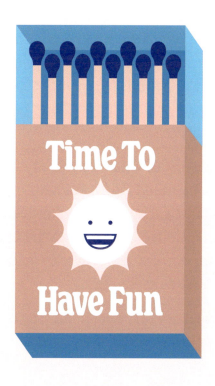

P. H.

Diagnoses:	**Autism, ADHD**
Age:	**52**
Diagnosed at:	**50**
Gender:	**Male; he/him**
Burnout type:	**Severe**

Two years ago, at age 50, I was diagnosed with ADHD. A decade earlier, I was starting a divorce and custody dispute, returning to college, earning a Bachelor's degree, and changing careers. When things settled down, the kids were moving away for college, and my job was not a good fit for me.

The stress of it all was too much. I "crashed". It wasn't like the depression I'd felt before, although I had no interest in doing anything. I felt drained—like someone had pulled the plug. Living alone and unemployed for six weeks, I slept for 16 to 20 hours a day. I had no appetite and lost 30 pounds in two months. I showered once a week, sometimes less. I couldn't pay bills, do laundry, shop for groceries, or manage my house.

In searching for help, my GP offered none. My family wasn't understanding, and I had no friends to ask for help. I stumbled across an article that mentioned autistic burnout and felt as though it was written for me. I mentioned the article to the psychologist I'd just started therapy with, who also happens to be on the short list of local doctors who evaluate adults for ASD.

Eventually, I returned to work, but I'm making only ⅓ of what I did before, because I've lost significant brain power. My financial troubles and anxiety have increased. I've lost more weight. I wake up exhausted and achy. At most, my energy level is 80% of what it was before—and often less.

At this point, it feels like I'm on a downward spiral, and that I'm only working myself into another burnout as I struggle just to get through each week.

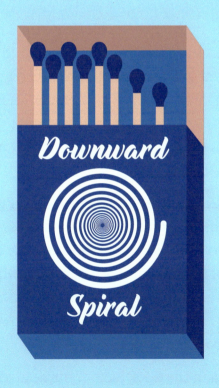

Janine K.

Diagnoses:	**Autism, ADHD (self-diagnosed)**
Age:	**58**
Diagnosed at:	**53**
Gender:	**Female; she/her**
Burnout type:	**Severe**

Like many late-diagnosed Gen-X women, I was taught that expressions of emotion, need, or want were wrong and bad, and that my safety depended upon everyone else's needs being met. Of course, this led to my inability to identify what I needed in the first place.

So, after a lifetime of trauma and alexithymia, I received a lifesaving autism diagnosis and was ready to begin to "find myself" when suddenly I found myself living as a full-time caregiver to my mother, whose memory was damaged by a massive stroke. It's been five years of reminding her each morning that I'm not angry with her (just because I don't know how to cheerfully modulate my voice before coffee as she asks me a dozen questions).

And—to add insult to injury—for the last year, I've been receiving treatment for cancer. At some point in the process of receiving treatment, I started to stutter for the first time in my life. I've also had several episodes of echolalia during meltdowns, which did very little for my reputation as an informed patient, so I bravely decided to tell my medical team I was autistic and, in general, have been receiving much better support as a result.

I'm aware that I'm in the thick haze of burnout as I write this, and frequently despair that it's here to stay, but I've begun identifying things that lift me out of that haze:

I joined a local writing group; I unapologetically call my (autistic) best friend, even when it means making dinner an hour later; I get outside into nature most days; I'm starting to drop my "capable" mask and ask for help.

And most importantly, I treat my wounded autistic self with "baby bird tenderness."

It helps.

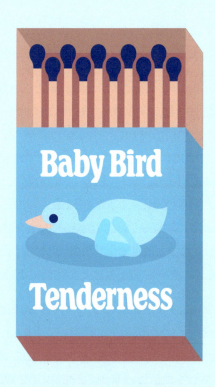

Russell McOrmond

Diagnoses:	**Autism, ADHD**
Age:	**56**
Diagnosed at:	**56**
Gender:	**Male; he/him**
Burnout type:	**Severe**

I have been part of the high-tech sector since my teens. In 2000, I heard that quite a bit of autism existed in the industry and I should look into it. I saw the ways autistic people were allegedly "defective", so I assumed that had nothing to do with me.

My mother's death in 2018 caused me to see a psychotherapist, and after seeing me for several months, I was asked if I had considered being autistic. I had doubts, partly because of the concept of an autistic mask. I was terrible at acting.

I never had regular job interviews and was brought into organizations because someone knew my skills and working methods. An exception occurred in 2018 when I was part of the merger of an organization I had been with for seven years. The new employer was a strict hierarchy with a strict chain of command, which saw job titles as exclusive jurisdiction. While I was focused on getting high-priority work done—working the same way I had at the previous employer—some people only saw me as violating a social hierarchy.

In the summer of 2022, I contracted Lyme Disease. Fatigue meant I didn't have the energy to mask—and thus, I finally accepted I had been masking. Accusations of being rude and condescending to allistic coworkers were made. I would respond with logic and data, but that only worsened things.

By the spring of 2023, I was accused of workplace harassment and placed on sick leave. That threw me into a full-on burnout, unable to manage regular life tasks. I lost all personal doubts I had about autism. When sick leave ran out at the end of the summer, I resigned—not seeing any room for me in that organization.

As I write this in the summer of 2024, I'm much better but still recovering. I believe learning I'm autistic and learning about **spoon theory** will help me avoid similar situations in the future. Learning about autism includes learning about allism.

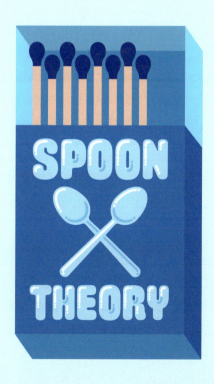

Rowan Mulder

Diagnoses:	**Autism, ADHD, alexithymia, major depression, generalized anxiety**
Age:	**31**
Diagnosed at:	**30**
Gender:	**Non-binary; they/them**
Burnout type:	**Severe**

My name is Rowan Mulder, and I am a 31-year-old nonbinary individual who uses they/them pronouns. I was diagnosed with autism, ADHD and alexithymia one year ago. I am also diagnosed with major depression and general anxiety. I have struggled with autistic burnout throughout my life. Currently, I am in the middle of a two-year severe burnout.

Before my burnout started, I was beginning my career as a Registered Nurse. Initially, I was very excited and threw everything into succeeding and excelling in my career. I was working 48 hours a week and taking classes to make the transition into my career smoother. I was in a constant state of overwhelm but heavily masking.

After eight months, I found myself depleted of all energy. All my time was spent recovering from my work week and neglecting self-care and home tasks. I was calling into work more frequently until I had to take a break from nursing altogether.

My main symptoms are chronic exhaustion, brain fog, increased sensory issues, skill regression, social withdrawal, executive dysfunction, depression, extreme anxiety/panic and a general feeling of overwhelm. I have also had an increase in meltdowns and their severity. At the height of my burnout, I had up to three meltdowns daily. Now, I am having one to two per week.

I had, and have, a lot of guilt and shame around the idea of resting and have tied my self-worth to productivity and the concept of "fixing myself". Consequently, I focused on recovering from burnout by "doing" instead of resting. Furthermore, my burnout was extended because I repeatedly found myself in the guilt and shame thought loops of needing to do more. Medication has done little to nothing for my symptoms.

Things that helped were reprocessing my trauma through the autistic lens, accommodating my sensory needs, decreasing demands, connecting with the autistic community, unmasking, and reading content by autistic or neurodivergent creators—for example, 'Unmasking Autism' by Devon Price.

I have been unable to return to my career; however, I have been working as a part-time direct support worker for eight months.

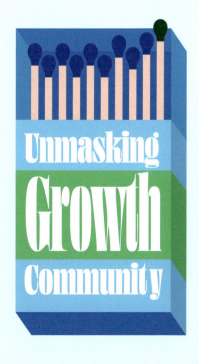

Alexander O.

Diagnoses:	**Autism, ADHD, alexithymia**
Age:	**27**
Diagnosed at:	**28**
Gender:	**Transmasculine; he/him**
Burnout type:	**Moderate**

In September 2023, I was working as an MSW intern at a private practice, immersed in the demands of learning a new role and working from home. I faced significant financial strain when my unemployment benefits were revoked, and I was unsure how to pay for everything. I tend to overwork myself and avoid how I'm feeling, but I knew I wasn't doing okay.

During this time, my grandmother passed away. I was very close to her, but even now, I couldn't tell you how I felt about it. It was almost as if my entire family fell apart while I tried to manage everything. Unfortunately, I had only three months left on my program, so there was absolutely no way I was going to withdraw.

I could tell I was at a tipping point. I was exhausted all the time, I wasn't being as kind as I should be to my loved ones, and I was still trying (and failing) to process my grief. My spouse's encouragement helped me realize I couldn't do it by myself anymore.

I had to start being honest with myself and with others. I found myself back in therapy (something I was ashamed to admit I needed), and this allowed me to process my grief. After my internship ended, I gave myself much-needed time.

I am still recovering from this period of my life, but I am also slowly starting to find my footing again. This speaks to me about the importance of prioritizing self-compassion in times of struggle. Resilience emerges in the face of adversity and reminds us of our strength and capacity for growth.

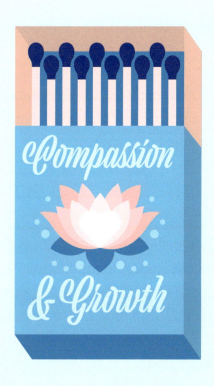

A. Rue

Diagnoses:	**Autism**
Age:	**40**
Diagnosed at:	**36**
Gender:	**Female; she/her**
Burnout type:	**Severe**

My name is A. Rue. Though I am a woman currently in my 40s, I'd say that burnout has been a part of the mental background noise since I was a teenager, cutting in and out over time.

College—in particular—had its share of frequent lows. I remember one occasion during class selection when I decided to increase my class load from four classes to five. I was laboring under the delusion that I wasn't working hard enough. While undertaking that schedule, I noticed a severe dip in my basic functioning. My stumbling way with words worsened. I'd forget basic vocabulary for the items I needed, from food to art supplies. (You haven't lived until you get into a staring match with someone trying to remember the word for both bamboo and paper.)

My grades also started to dip, which led to bouts of insomnia and my nerves burning with the anxiety of my "failure." I cut out basic functions to make up for the deficit. I couldn't figure out the defect in my programming for the life of me. Why could others handle an increased course load? Why was my life falling apart from the inclusion of one more obligation?

Eventually, I had to drink the poison that I couldn't handle it—one more class was too much. (Heck, four was already pushing me to my limits, not that I realized that until after graduation.) I dropped the extra class and reduced my expectations. My functionality returned over the year, and the world didn't end.

I wish my former self had made the connection that respecting one's limits isn't a sign of failure or against some internal set of made-up laws.

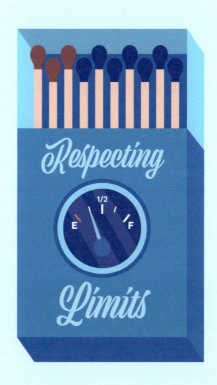

Nyx Lewis-Schmidt

Diagnoses:	**Autism, ADHD**
Age:	**27**
Diagnosed at:	**25**
Gender:	**Queer; they/them**
Burnout type:	**Severe**

When I graduated from university in 2019 and went straight into a full-time job, I was proud to be a productive member of society already working in my field. Two months later, however, I was falling back into the depression that had taken me out of university for a semester in 2017.

Conveniently, my employer shut down, leaving me suddenly without a job, just as I was reaching the point where I thought I would have to quit.

This situation was the start of a years-long cycle. I would get a job and work for a month or two. Then, my mental health would begin to spiral into depression, exhaustion, and panic attacks. I would quit the job, slowly start to recover, try a new job, spiral, quit, rinse, repeat.

Eventually, I was diagnosed autistic, and I began to understand that what I was experiencing was autistic burnout—but the realization came too late to save me from the severe burnout I am still living in.

I have accepted that I may never be able to work a consistent job. I deal with severe fatigue and brain fog alongside my chronic pain. I can manage one or two tasks on a good day, like taking out the garbage or washing dishes. On a bad day, it's hard even to feed myself.

I'm lucky to have an amazing and understanding wife (also AuDHD) who supports me, along with help from our parents. I do what I can and try not to judge myself for what I can't, but that part is hard. It's hard to remind myself that I have intrinsic value and don't have to be productive to be worthy of existing or being happy.

But we do deserve to be happy. We are worthy. And we deserve rest.

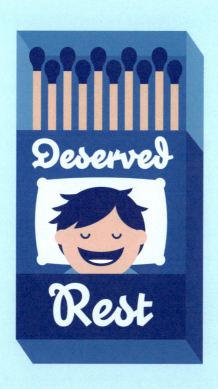

Susan

Diagnoses:	**Autism, ADHD, alexithymia**
Age:	**30**
Diagnosed at:	**29**
Gender:	**Genderfluid; she/her**
Burnout type:	**Severe**

I was born in Paris, France, but mostly grew up in Brooklyn, New York. Both of my parents are Middle Eastern immigrants. I identify as Mizrahi Jewish.

I have a Bachelor's in Sociology but no other certification or license. I was employed on and off as an educator. I moved out from my father's home in June 2018. I have moved three more times since then. From June 2018 until July 2023, I had significantly more built-in support and was functioning much better.

The factors that resulted in Severe Burnout were the following:

1. Stress related to increased responsibilities for the first time;

2. Job stress, including bullying from the lead teacher due to her inability to manage her stress. Also, problems that generally happen periodically had happened in rapid succession;

3. Several tragedies that happened to family and friends;

4. Some virtual support, but an overall lack of consistent, in-person friendships and community that feel safe and non-judgmental.

My official breaking point was Friday, December 22nd. Up to then, I had more miniature versions of crisis from which I still seemed to bounce back. I was declining in my functioning but still showing up to my job early and leaving late so that I could complete my work.

I got better at identifying and understanding my warning signs. To prevent burnout, I am looking into applying for disability benefits, supportive housing, and food assistance, so that I can support myself while going to a therapy facility multiple days a week. I worked through a neurodivergent-friendly DBT workbook and other worksheets related to autistic burnout.

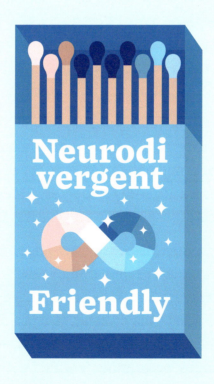

Adrienne S.

Diagnoses:	**Autism, ADHD, alexithymia**
Age:	**65**
Diagnosed at:	**62**
Gender:	**Female; she/her**
Burnout type:	**Incidental**

I'm a very late-diagnosed autistic. I spent most of my life not understanding certain experiences, including autistic burnout. I remember just before my 32nd birthday, my mother called to tell me my grandfather was receiving hospice care. The expectation was that he would live only a few days. I flew home, and panicked I might miss the chance to say goodbye. As relatives arrived throughout the week, my grandfather hung on. With the anticipation of losing someone I cherished, I felt weaker and more disoriented each day.

My birthday came; my whole body ached, and I had horrible abdominal pains. I asked my brother to take me to a doctor, hoping it'd bring peace of mind. The doctor found nothing specific but advised me to follow up with my doctor back home. My anxiety escalated. When I returned to my parents' house, I collapsed into bed, craving silence and solitude.

At dinnertime, my mother knocked on my door. She'd ordered Chinese food for my birthday. Feeling immovable, I told her I couldn't eat. She gritted her teeth and, true to her stiff-upper-lip upbringing, insisted I get up and "just pretend." Despite feeling wholly dysregulated at the situation's absurdity, I complied—knowing that she, too, was torn. Besides, pretending is what I did best—a skill that consistently propped me up, as it did again when my grandfather passed away later that night.

Being recently diagnosed, I'm still learning the signs that I'm heading for burnout and when to say no. I find meditation, breathing exercises, journaling, and walking in nature helpful.

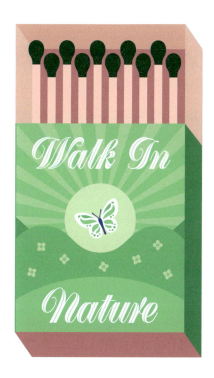

Eva Silvertant

Diagnoses:	**Autism, ADHD, alexithymia**
Age:	**35**
Diagnosed at:	**25**
Gender:	**Trans-female; she/her**
Burnout type:	**Severe (2022) to moderate (now)**

In 2022, I went through a prolonged period of daily emotional crisis. I experienced occupational burnout from pushing myself too hard for too long with my work, autistic burnout from trying to handle responsibilities and social tasks beyond what I could manage—not longterm and in a sustainable way, anyway—and depression due to other life circumstances.

As a result, I could not work or fulfill any of my responsibilities. I was virtually unable to perform my daily tasks for Embrace Autism. Every day, I would tell myself that today was the day I would meet some of my responsibilities, but I just couldn't.

It took me months before I could admit to any of my colleagues that I had not been working much—too ashamed to tell them how much I struggled; and I probably couldn't quite admit it to myself either.

When colleagues asked whether I finished a project I was supposed to do, I would tell them I was working on it, and that I would get it done soon. That was never a lie; I *was* working on it, and I really thought I would get it done soon. But I never got as much done as I thought I would. Every day, I thought I was going to be able to manage, and then just didn't. I would see a lot of time go by and be frustrated that I had so little to show for it; that I wasn't able to finish any projects.

Even though it wasn't my fault that I was struggling so severely, I couldn't help but take my dysfunction personally and think of myself as a failure—lazy even. I felt too ashamed to fully acknowledge my condition and seek help for it. My shame and guilt around not getting things done was eating me up inside.

I used to cry every night under the stars while listening to music that intensified my emotions. I know it sounds dramatic, but I would wallow in self-pity and self-hatred. I think I became addicted to **oxytocin** and **endorphins** released from all the crying. **Dopamine** and oxytocin are released during catharsis, which makes you feel good—but then you seek that relief again.

I was a mess, and I think there were several contributing factors:

1. I began my gender transition in 2021. While this brought me a profound sense of happiness as I could finally live authentically without hiding my true self, I also had to face the impact of hormonal influences on my emotions, thoughts, and behaviors. It affected me more deeply than I had anticipated, leading to the experience of much stronger emotions.

   On the positive side, it helped me address long-standing traumas that I had been unaware of for years by reducing my alexithymia. However, this process was far from easy, quick, or pleasant. During this time, I found myself highly emotionally reactive, likening it to experiencing a second puberty. The early stages of transitioning are often described this way, as we must learn to navigate new emotional experiences and ways of relating.

2. Before undergoing transition, I was primarily focused on my ideas and intellectual contributions. I would derive most of my validation and sense of worth from writing and sharing my

knowledge and insights. However, after the hormonal changes, I became less solitary and more focused on relationships. Suddenly, my validation and sense of self-worth came from my relationships and what I meant to my friends rather than my intellectual accomplishments. This adjustment was quite challenging, and I had to essentially rediscover myself and find new coping mechanisms.

3. I believe that my ADHD significantly worsened my struggles with coping mechanisms. My anxiety was so intense that it led to a lot of procrastination. And the more I put things off, the less I achieved, and the less validation I received. As a result, my self-worth decreased, and my self-esteem suffered. Along the way, I realized that while I may not have much self-esteem, I rely on what some call 'other-esteem'—meaning that my sense of worth is derived from the approval of others rather than an intrinsic sense of self-worth.

4. I have also struggled with substance use disorder (cannabis and tobacco) since I was 21. Initially, it had a positive influence, as it helped me be okay with putting down my work now and then and actually take a rest; it allowed me to enjoy watching movies and series without getting bored. Before then, only work would really captivate mend give me enough stimulation. Besides extra cognitive stimulation, it also allowed me to suppress my sensory stimulation and cope better with my anxiety. But along the way, this balance of work and off-time became severely skewed, and I became dependent in order to cope with my anxiety, and to help with self-regulation.

And I feel proud about the fact that I have been sober since 6 January 2023!

With all the aforementioned factors, I found myself in a spiral of diminishing self-esteem and motivation, making it increasingly difficult to get out of burnout. I thought something had fundamentally snapped in me and that there was no chance of ever recovering. Rest didn't help because it reinforced my perception of myself as lazy, broken, and worthless.

What really locked me into place and prevented any progress was how self-critical and downright cruel I was to myself, constantly comparing myself to what I used to be able to do. I had a strong work ethic before, so I couldn't understand why everything suddenly required more energy and motivation than I could muster.

Joining a virtual substance use program ultimately helped me recover. I found a sense of belonging and a community by uniting with others with a common purpose. I no longer felt alone in my struggle. Despite facing challenges, knowing that I wasn't alone and receiving the emotional support I needed started to turn things around for me.

We would celebrate minor accomplishments. I think that's very important. Sure, my accomplishments were minuscule compared to what I used to be able to do. But you know what? They were still accomplishments! It was more than nothing at all. That's progress. That's not something we should diminish, even when the progress may seem insignificant or too slow.

The more of these minor accomplishments I was able to acknowledge and celebrate, the more motivation and energy I got for the next accomplishment. They could be as little as showing up for virtual codependency meetings. But gradually I learned to better self-regulate; I learned to maintain emotional sobriety. I stuck to healthier routines, I picked up my walking routine again, and along the way, my accomplishments incrementally became bigger.

This was 1.5 years ago now. I felt I significantly recovered from my burnout. I was doing things again! I was more active and more functional. And all of that is true. But some months ago, I took a burnout test, and I was quite shocked by the results. It showed I was still significantly burned out. I started crying because I realized it was true. Yes, I'm still burned out. I came a long way and healed more than I deemed possible, and I'm immensely grateful for that. But I still have a way to go...

I feel more or less recovered from occupational burnout, but autistic burnout remains. I can be functional and do some work, but responding to messages and emails is still very overwhelming. I still find those things very difficult to manage. Maintaining a conversation online with anyone except for my best friend is even more challenging. Maintaining an ongoing conversation feels like too much responsibility to me right now. I strongly desire to be more social because relationships are much more fulfilling to me now than they used to be. But right now, the effort required to maintain communication with more than a very selected few people is just more than I can handle.

But I'm hopeful. I'm about to start therapy with someone with AuDHD like me, who specializes in anxiety. I think they can help me get better coping mechanisms to deal with anxiety and help me overcome my postponing behaviour. I don't think I will be cured a few weeks into my therapy. But just as before, I think I will experience incremental progress. Progress may be slow, and that's okay.

I may or may not become as functional and driven as I used to be, and that's fine. I went in overdrive for too many years anyway, and I need to stop comparing myself with who I used to be and what I used to be able to do. I need to show self-compassion and acceptance of the things that are beyond my control.

All I can do is make the best out of my current situation and capabilities. Achieving perfection and optimal performance shouldn't be my goals anymore because they aren't sustainable or achievable; I'm only human. I need to find an optimal balance—a way of living that is both functional and worthwhile. And I need to keep celebrating even minor accomplishments. Progress and growth rather than perfection should be my goals.

You know, producing this book often seemed like an insurmountable task. And I did beat myself up a lot about what I felt I should have accomplished in a day but didn't. But I did do some work every day.

And the fruit of my (incremental) labour eventually became a significant accomplishment. I'm really proud of what I've done, and of my progress in my recovery.

You will get there, too! You're not alone in this...

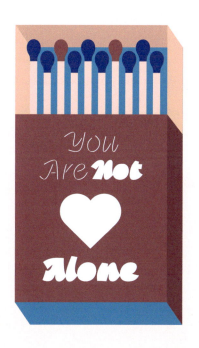 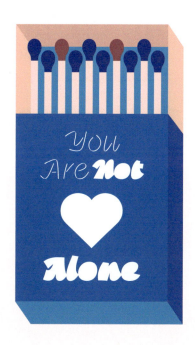

Patient Handouts

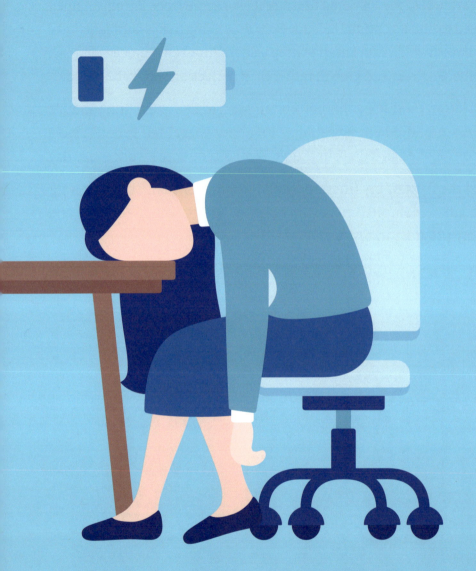

On the following pages are some supplementary materials such as forms that you can print out and use. The forms are also provided as separate files, which may be easier to print.

Table of Contents
Patient Handouts

Energy Inventory Instructions

- Use the left column to describe activities or experiences from today or yesterday which you experienced as draining (blue form) or energizing (green form).

- Rate the activity/experience on a four-point scale (how draining or energizing was the activity/experience?). Reserve four points for the activities/experiences that completely drained you that day, or completely rejuvenated you.

- Use the right column to add additional information for your doctor (or for yourself) for more context.

- Add the date so that you can track your energy loss or acquisition over time. That way, you may me able to observe patterns and/or see progress.

Symptom Sheet for Your Medical Practitioner

Describe your symptom. Print out a new sheet for each symptom.

General description

Symptom: _____

Where do you notice the symptom? _____

Is it constant or intermittent? _____

When does the symptom occur? _____

How long does it last when it happens? _____

Does it radiate anywhere (does it extend beyond the main area)? ___

_____

Severity:* _____

*Use the severity scale on the right page. Bring this page to your pracitioner.

What is the symptom interfering with in your life? _____

_____

What other symptoms do you have with it? _____

_____

Evolution of symptoms

When did the symptom start? _____

Has the symptom been getting better or worse? _____

How quickly has the symptom been getting better or worse? _____

_____

What makes the symptom better or worse (e.g., food, sleep, stress)?

_____

Explored treatments

What have you tried to make it better? _____

Medications? _____

Supplements? _____

Physical therapy? _____

Severity Scale

This is probably the most difficult thing for an autistic to describe, and it leads to the healthcare practitioner not understanding the severity of the symptom.

It is best to describe how it is affecting your life; you can also use the scale below and tell your doctor both the description and the number to indicate the severity.

Score	Meaning
1	**Symptom is very mild**—barely noticeable. Most of the time, you don't think about it.
2	**Minor symptom.** It's annoying. You may have a strong symptom now and then.
3	**Noticeable symptom.** It may distract you, but you can get used to it.
4	**Moderate symptom.** Wen involved in an activity, you can ignore the symptom for a while. But it is still distracting.
5	**Moderately strong symptom.** You can't ignore it for more than a few minutes. But, you can still work or do some social activities with effort.
6	**Moderately stronger symptom.** You avoid some of your normal daily activities. You have trouble concentrating.
7	**Strong symptom.** It keeps you from doing normal activities—including work and socializing.
8	**Very strong symptom.** It's hard to do anything at all.
9	**Symptom that is very hard to tolerate.** You can't carry on a conversation.
10	**Worst symptom possible.** It is unbearable.

Energy Inventory

Activities & Experiences That <u>Take</u> Energy

Activities/experiences	Rating	Comments
	○○○○	
	○○○○	
	○○○○	
	○○○○	
	○○○○	
	○○○○	
	○○○○	
	○○○○	
	○○○○	
	○○○○	
	○○○○	
	○○○○	
	○○○○	
	○○○○	
	○○○○	
	○○○○	
	○○○○	
	○○○○	
	○○○○	

● = mild   ●● = moderate   ●●● = significant   ●●●● = catastrophic

Energy Inventory

Activities/experiences	Rating	Comments
	○○○○	
	○○○○	
	○○○○	
	○○○○	
	○○○○	
	○○○○	
	○○○○	
	○○○○	
	○○○○	
	○○○○	
	○○○○	
	○○○○	
	○○○○	
	○○○○	
	○○○○	
	○○○○	
	○○○○	
	○○○○	
	○○○○	
	○○○○	
	○○○○	

Activities & Experiences That <u>Give</u> Energy

● = mild   ●● = moderate   ●●● = significant   ●●●● = catastrophic

Energy Inventory

Activities & Experiences That <u>Take</u> Energy

Activities/experiences	Rating	Comments
Socializing	●●●○	Very draining depending on the person
Change	●●●○	Unexpected changes can be really disruptive
Making a mistake	●○○○	
Sensory sensitivity	●●●○	
Daily living skills	●●○○	
Coping with anxiety	●●●○	My anxiety throughout the day can be very draining as it often keeps me preoccupied
Overanalyzing social performance	●●○○	
Sensitivity to other people's moods	●○○○	
Being teased or excluded	●●○○	
Crowds	●●○○	
Filling in forms	●●●○	Multi-page forms tend to be really daunting
Responding to emails	●●●○	I mostly avoid emails; they are too draining and anxiety-inducing
Dealing with government agencies	●●○○	
Meltdown & shutdown	●●●●	Meltdowns disrupt my entire day
Perceived injustice	●●○○	
Certain people	●●●●	Some people I have to avoid or I get drained
Making dinner	●●●○	
Doing laundry	●●○○	
Cleaning the house	●●●○	Sometimes it's just too much to handle
Doing groceries	●●●○	Logistics of getting ingredients + sensory stimulation
Feeding the pets	●○○○	

● = mild ●● = moderate ●●● = significant ●●●● = catastrophic

Energy Inventory

Activities & Experiences That <u>Give</u> Energy		
Activities/experiences	**Rating**	**Comments**
Solitude	●●●○	I need a lot of alone time to restore
Special interest	●●●○	I can get really lost in my special interests in a good way; it can restore my energy
Physical activity	●○○○	
Pets/animals	●●○○	Being with my pets and cuddling them is energizing; but their needs are draining
Nature	●●●○	
Playing computer games	●●●○	Computer games offer me a sense of escape from the daily demands
Meditation	●○○○	Can help a little bit, but I have to be in the right head space for it to work
Mindfulness	●○○○	
Caring for others	●○○○	Can give some energy if things go well, but I often don't know how I can help
Nutrition/food	●●○○	
Sleep	●●●●	Can be fully restorative, provided I don't go to bed angry or upset
Reading a book	●●○○	
Focus on mental health	●○○○	Can help. but can also be draining
Vacation day	●●●●	A day without responsibilities or (social) demands can be fully restorative
Browse information online	●●○○	
Certain people	●●●○	A few people in my life give me energy; they motivate me and offer support
Listening to music	●●○○	
Listening to audio book	●○○○	Not as restorative as listening to music, as it requires more of my attention and focus
Watching a movie/series	●●●○	
Creative pursuit	●●●○	Drawing can be really therapeutic
Gardening	●○○○	

● = mild ●● = moderate ●●● = significant ●●●● = catastrophic   © 2024 Embrace Autism

Explaining Autistic Burnout to Friends and Family

What is Autistic Burnout?

Autistic burnout is a medical condition caused by spending too much time in stressful environments where an autistic individual cannot keep up with the demands.

Autistic burnout is not the same thing as job burnout (officially called 'occupational burnout'); unlike job burnout, autistic burnout can be caused by many things in the (social) environment.

The research shows that burnout can be due to:

- **Social demands** (e.g., I have too many social events, my environment requires me to perform social norms, I am in a relationship with someone who doesn't understand autism)
- **Sensory demands** (e.g., my environment is not sensory-friendly)
- **Daily life demands** (e.g., I have too many errands and administrative tasks)
- **Insufficient support** (e.g., at work, school, and/or at home)

It's important to understand that my burnout isn't caused by being autistic. It's caused by **not having my autistic needs met** while living in a neurotypical society.

The Impacts of Autistic Burnout

Autistic burnout impacts me in the following ways:

- I may "look more autistic".

- I am not able to mask/camouflage as much.

- I am having a harder time communicating with speech.

- I am feeling more emotionally dysregulated (e.g., I am experiencing more meltdowns/shutdowns).

- My mental health is worse (e.g., depression and anxiety).

- I am more suicidal (e.g., thinking about suicide, planning to attempt suicide).

- I am often/constantly physically and cognitively exhausted and overwhelmed.

- I am more forgetful, I am having more trouble paying attention, I have brain fog.

- I can't keep up with my work, it's taking me longer to process things and complete tasks.

- I am having trouble organizing my time.

- I am more affected by changes in my routine and unexpected things that arise.

- My sensory sensitivities are more intense.

- Other: _____

The way I am feeling fluctuates from day-to-day. Some days I may have more energy and feel more like my baseline, but that doesn't necessarily mean that I've recovered or that I'm faking the severity of my experiences.

Things I Need for Recovery

The following is a list of the things that I need in order to recover from autistic burnout:

- I need to withdraw from people and social events (it's not personal!).
- I need to reduce my workload.
- I need to take a break from work/school.
- I need to spend more time alone in my room undisturbed.
- I need to take a break from communicating with speech.
- I need to make time to engage in my special interests.
- I need help creating a suicide safety plan.
- Other: _____

It may take me months or even years to recover. Please be patient!

Reducing the Chance of Burnout

In order to reduce the chance that I experience autistic burnout in the future, I need the following:

- To change how I work or go to school (e.g., part-time, quit).
- More support around daily tasks (e.g., groceries, paying bills).
- Accommodations at work/school.
- A routine that allows me to engage in my special interests.
- A safe space where I can escape from sensory demands.
- To find a therapist who understands autism.
- To meet more autistic people and grow my community.
- Other: _____

Because my burnout is caused by environmental factors, I need to make significant changes in my life to ensure that my needs are met.

Click the link below to download a package with all the forms and other materials from the Patient Handouts section—as well as several Autistic Burnout posters you can print out:

Embrace-Autism.com/autistic-burnout-download

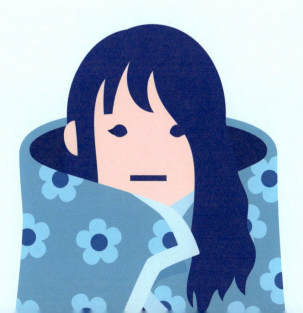